Three Great Teachers
of Osteopathy

Three Great Teachers of Osteopathy

Lessons We Learned from
Drs. Becker, Fulford, and Wales

Edited by Rachel E. Brooks, MD

StillnessPress

Stillness Press, LLC
Portland, Oregon
www.stillnesspress.com

Edited by Rachel E. Brooks, M.D.
Book and cover design by Lubosh Cech *luboshcech.com*

ISBN   979-8-9875675-0-0 (Hardcover Edition)
ISBN   978-0-9675851-6-1 (Softcover Edition)
ISBN   978-0-9675851-7-8 (eBook Edition)

Stillness Press books are available at www.stillnesspress.com

*When you come home to yourself others
can find themselves in you.*

Handbook for the Evolving Heart
through
Frank Coppieters, PhD

Contents

Introduction

Rachel Brooks

I am a storyteller. I guess I always have been, but I only came to truly understand that about myself in the process of working on this book. I have always wondered with amusement how the young person that I was in college, who had thought she might be destined to be a social worker or lawyer or even a historian, instead decided to become a medical doctor. It seemed an abrupt and inexplicable leap at the time, but I am so very glad that I did. I see now that whatever course I had taken in life, storytelling would naturally have had to be a part of that work.

I am captivated by the human story. I experience people's stories as being one of my important teachers – providing insight about so many aspects of life. In my practice, I am grateful for the stories my patients share with me, and I often tell stories to them when offering guidance, reassurance, and even hard truths. In my teaching, stories punctuate every presentation I make, and the stories told to me by my osteopathic teachers are a treasure I carry with me. Yes, I am a storyteller – and so, upon reflection, it seems natural that I initiated this project of collecting stories.

While the essence of osteopathy is taught hand-to-hand, there is also a long and deep tradition of osteopathic inspiration and wisdom being imparted through the words and deeds of the teachers and elders of their day. Sometimes this teaching is widely broadcast and is widely known; but often it is imparted person-to-person. Whatever the means of transmission, what each learner takes away is generally as much about the learner as it is about the teacher. In this book of "lessons we learned," I strived to capture a unique view of the teachings of these great teachers by focusing on those who received their lessons.

The Teachers and the Stories

Why These Three Teachers

The stories in this book are about Drs. Rollin Becker, Robert Fulford, and Anne Wales – three remarkable practitioners and teachers of osteopathy in the cranial field (OCF) who were personally inspired by their connection with its developer, Dr. William G. Sutherland. Why just these three when there were many other important figures in the development and teaching of OCF? One major reason is that they lived long enough and taught widely enough to directly influence many of the current "elders" in the cranial osteopathic profession. These three are also the ones I personally had the most significant contact with. I was extremely fortunate to have had personal relationships with Rollin Becker and Anne Wales over many years, and I had encountered Robert Fulford in many courses.

Beginning in the 1990s, because of the close connection I was known to have with Dr. Becker, I was often called upon to give lectures about him and his teachings. And, not surprisingly, these presentations were filled with stories. Afterwards, some of those in the audience would invariably come up to me and tell me their own stories of experiences with Dr. Becker: stories of insights gained and of lives changed. These same people would often also tell me stories about Dr. Wales and Dr. Fulford.

Three Great Teachers of Osteopathy – An Overview

These three great teachers of osteopathy – Drs. Becker, Fulford, and Wales – were born in the first decade of the twentieth century and entered osteopathic college in the 1920s and 30s. Each of their lives was transformed by meeting Dr. William G. Sutherland, the developer of osteopathy in the cranial field (OCF), in the 1940s. At that time Sutherland was in his 70's and they were in their 30's and 40's. This timeline afforded each of them a decade or less to learn from Dr. Sutherland before he died in 1954.

Drs. Becker and Wales both developed a warm personal relationship with Dr. Sutherland. They were particularly devoted to his teaching and became part of his teaching faculty. Dr. Fulford studied with Dr. Sutherland but also had strong connections with other teachers in this field. How they each spoke about Dr. Sutherland's character also revealed something about themselves. Anne would often simply say: "Dr. Sutherland was the most mature person I had ever met." This was a deeply meaningful statement from Anne, expressing both gratitude and admiration. It was not only a reflection on his presence but also on the way he handled situations. Robert gave this description: "Dr. Sutherland was a quiet man whose radiance spoke of a tremendous vitality of spirit. In his eyes flickered a constant, subtle, inspiring light. When his vision took you in and those eyes narrowed, you could feel that he was gazing not at your physical body, but at your inner being." (*Dr. Fulford's Touch of Life*, 188) Rollin once shared: "William Garner Sutherland was a quiet man, the most beautiful man I ever met. Every one of you would love him. If you saw a picture of him, it would be like falling in love with your spiritual teacher or someone very special. He just had that kind of presence." (*The Stillness of Life*, 5)

All three of these teachers played an important role in keeping the teaching of OCF alive in the years after Sutherland's death. There was very limited interest from the osteopathic profession in these teachings during the 1950s and 60s, and the perseverance of all who carried on the teaching was essential. In the mid-70s and 80s, there was a growing interest in "wholistic medicine" and the teaching of OCF began to expand among a more receptive audience.

Over the decades, each of these teachers carried this work forward in their own way. They were three individuals whose way of practicing OCF was distinct and unique to who they were. What they had in common included a deep dedication to their work; a commitment to continual growth; a lifelong willingness to teach; and, at the core of their being, they had a strong and profoundly clear presence.

For me, an example of their unique ways of being was in how their clear presence manifested when they were treating. Whatever else they were do-ing in a treatment or whatever approach they were using, my sense was that they each had a distinct state of being that predominated. My perceptions were: Anne Wales was extraordinarily grounded; she was connected to the forces of earth; Rollin Becker was deeply attuned to Stillness; he sat im-mersed in a field of that all-pervasive potential energy; Robert Fulford had a living connectedness to the universal energies; he embodied an awareness of the energies of Life and Love.

A mutual respect existed among these three. They did not necessarily agree upon all things related to OCF, but there was respect; and between Becker and Wales there was also a longtime friendship. One representation of this respect is the clear memory I have of Dr. Becker at the last cranial conference he attended in 1988. During one lecture session, I watched him edging his way forward in the lecture hall with a hand cupped behind his ear to better hear what Dr. Fulford had to say from the podium.

The Stories in This Book

The stories that make up this book are wide-ranging and varied. Some of the stories collected come from people who encountered these teachers when they were young students or early in their practice life; others were fully formed practitioners with many years of experience under their belts. Some of the stories arise from those who had just a single interaction with one of these teachers. Other stories come from those who had long rela-tionships with one or more of them over many years.

Each person who shared a story for this book was inspired, in ways small or large. For some, the lesson learned brought some helpful insight, while for others the experience was life changing. In many instances, the lesson learned was clear from the start, in other instances the meaning and value of the lesson only became apparent over many years.

All the stories are told from the perspective of the one receiving the teaching. Whatever the teacher might have meant or intended at the time, this is a book of the lessons *we* learned. The stories are not intended to provide a personal biography or summation of the teachings of these three teachers, however they do provide a view into the nature and thinking of these important osteopaths.

The earliest stories in this book take place around the mid-1970s. At that time, these three teachers would have been in osteopathic practice roughly between 35 and 50 years. The reader will find that there are many remarkable stories in this book, and that is due, in large measure, to the fact that they were remarkable people who were remarkably committed to what they did. It is also true that the storytellers who received these lessons benefited by receiving them when these great teachers had garnered the wisdom and skill that grows with age and long experience.

The stories of Dr. Becker continue through to 1988 when he last taught at a course before he became disabled at the age of 78. Dr. Fulford gave his last lecture presentation in 1997 just six days before he died at the age of 91. Dr. Wales continued to teach groups, large and small, into the early 2000s when she was over 100 years old.

Share Your Story

Upon reading this book, I am confident that those of you who knew these teachers will have stories of your own to share. If you do, please share them for an anticipated second volume. In addition to more stories about Drs. Becker, Fulford, and Wales, I want to expand the collection to include stories of any of the other students of Dr. Sutherland.

To share a story – please contact Rachel Brooks, MD through:
"Share a Story" at www.stillnesspress.com

Osteopathy and Osteopathy in the Cranial Field

*(A brief description is offered here to give some background
information and context for the stories in this book.)*

Osteopathy and Dr. Still

Following a period of intense study into the nature of health and healing, a frontier doctor in the late nineteenth century, Andrew Taylor Still,
developed the science of osteopathy. At the core of his teaching was the
insight that the ills that befell living creatures involved some impairment in
the free flow of the material and non-material (energetic) elements within
the body, thereby impeding the normal, ever-present process of renewal,
regeneration, and re-formation.

Dr. Still's osteopathy was deeply rooted in anatomy, with a focus on
details both large and small. He studied and taught the intricate details and
function not only of macro structures like the bones and organs, but also
the finest elements of the nerves, fluids, and fascia.

Melding science and spirituality, Dr. Still also delved into the mysteries
of the life process. He sought to recognize and understand the forces that
create and sustain life – forces that are essential to health and healing.

Based on all of his understanding, Dr. Still developed a treatment approach that used manual contacts together with a knowledge of the living
mechanism to allow the restoration of normal, healthy functioning.

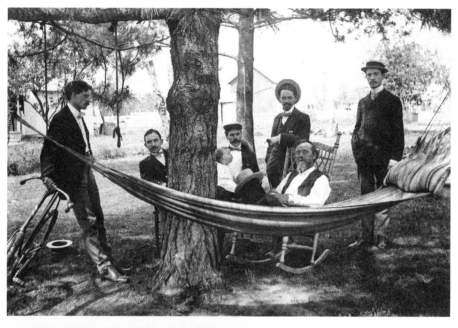

American School of Osteopathy students visiting A.T. Still at Morris Farm, circa 1900.

Museum of Osteopathic Medicine, Kirksville, MO [cat#: 1985.1003.25].

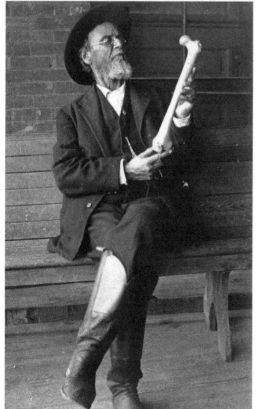

A.T. Still examining a femur.

Museum of Osteopathic Medicine, Kirksville, MO [cat#: 1995.29.06].

The Cranial Concept and Dr. Sutherland

In the first half of the twentieth century, William Garner Sutherland extended Still's osteopathy into the *cranial field* through his own flash of insight into the inherent mechanisms in the body. He perceived by direct experience that there were subtle, meaningful movements involving the cranial bones, central nervous system, cerebrospinal fluid, with associated movements of the sacrum and membranous structures. Working with this insight, that he called "the cranial concept," he observed that these subtle movements and the forces that created them were a crucial expression of healthy functioning.

Dr. Sutherland went on to develop a treatment approach that engaged these subtle, inherent movements and forces to address the restrictions and limitations impeding the full expression of health. Because this approach was first applied to diagnose and treat problems in the cranial mechanism, it became known as "cranial osteopathy" or "osteopathy in the cranial field." However, these subtle physiologic expressions of life are present throughout the body and the same treatment approaches can be used wherever limitations are found. And so, while it continues to be known as "cranial" osteopathy, it really is, and always has been, simply a part of the greater field of osteopathy.

The Primary Respiratory Mechanism and Life Forces

One term in the cranial concept that is frequently used in this book is the *primary respiratory mechanism* (PRM). Dr. Sutherland coined this term to describe the primary features that he observed with his hands-on sensory contact: the individual anatomical features of the craniosacral mechanism moving in a physiologic rhythmic, tide-like (cyclic) mechanism of motion. This motion is *involuntary* and is a fundamental expression of life. It has perceivable diagnostic characteristics that include vitality, amplitude, and direction which can be impacted by osteopathic treatment. Dr. Sutherland understood the mechanism's rhythmic, involuntary motion to be a *primary* form of respiration – it being essential to physiological functioning, including the respiration of the lungs.

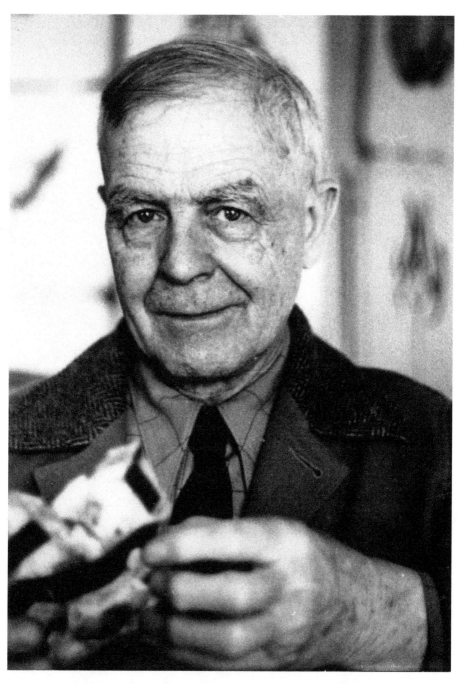

Dr. Sutherland teaching in St. Peter, Minnesota, January 1945. A class photo shows 12 participants in attendance (including Rollin Becker).

Although Dr. Sutherland defined the PRM in connection with the movement of specific anatomic structures, he always emphasized that the inherent life forces being manifested were of the greatest import. Sutherland spoke of these forces as the *Breath of Life* and *Potency* – forces that can be experienced but that are not yet truly understood; forces which motivate the primary respiration of living things.

In recent decades, modern science has shown many of Still and Sutherland's key findings and fundamental concepts to be true. They were visionaries and extraordinarily keen observers and thinkers.

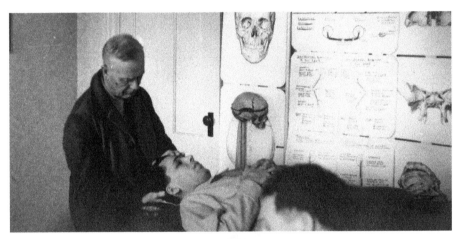

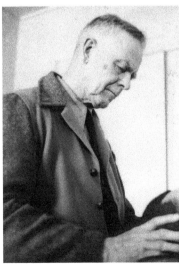
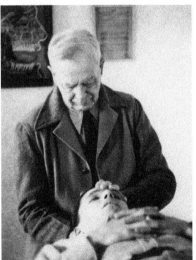

Four photos of Dr. Sutherland teaching in St. Peter, Minnesota, January 1945.

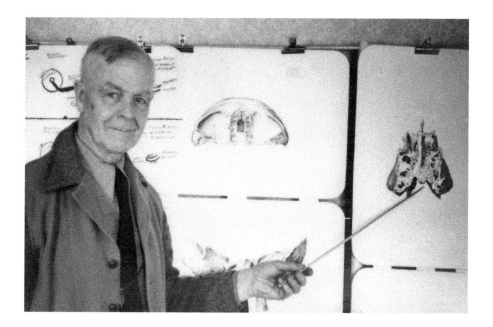

Terminology Usage

Given that the stories in this book are told based on the understanding of each storyteller, you will find variations in how the term primary respiratory mechanism (PRM) is used. In some instances, the usage will closely match Sutherland's definition and in others it might be used in a way that reflects a broader or more generalized meaning or simply a less precisely defined one; and sometimes reference is made simply to "the mechanism." There are also terms used that are considered synonymous with the PRM, including the *craniosacral mechanism* and the *involuntary mechanism*.

Organizations

Two US organizations dedicated to the teaching of osteopathy in the cranial field are mentioned frequently in this book. They are the Osteopathic Cranial Academy (OCA) and the Sutherland Cranial Teaching Foundation, Inc (SCTF). The OCA is a professional membership organization that was established in 1947 by members of the osteopathic profession interested in establishing professional support and ongoing education in the cranial field. The SCTF is an educational foundation established in 1953 by Dr. Sutherland and senior members of his teaching faculty to help perpetuate his teachings.

Rollin E. Becker, DO

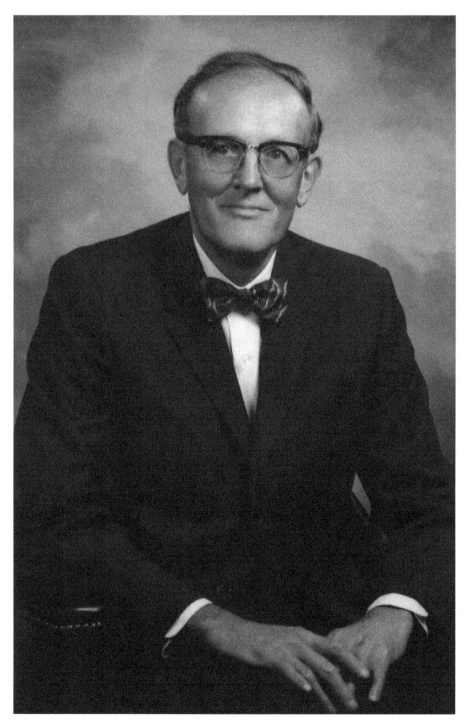

Rollin Becker, a photographic portrait. Another version of this photo exists in which the lower portion has been cropped out. Dr. Becker told his son that he preferred the one that showed his hands.

Rollin E. Becker, DO
(1910 – 1996)

Rollin Becker was born into an osteopathic family in Kirksville, Missouri. At the time of his birth, his father, Arthur Becker, DO, was a member of the teaching faculty at the American School of Osteopathy under the guidance of its founder, Andrew Taylor Still. Although the family later moved on from Kirksville, Rollin returned there for his osteopathic education, graduating in 1934.

Dr. Becker possessed a spiritual orientation throughout his life – beginning with influences from his parents, who held spiritual beliefs without a particular religious affiliation. His interests and explorations in this area were wide-ranging, and he read books on spiritual teachings in both western and eastern traditions. And while Rollin never maintained a specific spiritual practice or affiliation with a particular teaching, his life and his osteopathic work were guided by spiritual principles. The core of his beliefs was of a direct connection with the Infinite that exists in all of life, and the ability each person has to experience and live in that Presence.

After some years in general practice, Dr. Becker felt a need to understand osteopathy on a deeper level than he had been taught. He began with a more in-depth study of Dr. Still's teachings. In Still's writings he found a wealth of ideas for exploration as well as the specific guidance he needed to deepen his osteopathic experience. In 1944, Dr. Becker met William G. Sutherland and was deeply inspired by the man and his teachings. Rollin had both a great love for Sutherland and a devotion to developing his own understanding and skills.

In 1948, he became part of Sutherland's teaching faculty, and he continued that dedication to preserving and teaching osteopathy in the cranial field for decades after Sutherland's death in 1954. Dr. Becker was closely affiliated with the Sutherland Cranial Teaching Foundation and served as its president from 1962-1979.

The guidance of both Still and Sutherland led Dr. Becker to learn from the most authoritative source available – the living forces present within the living body. He became a ceaseless observer, continually seeking an answer to the question: What is "health" and what is the most efficient and effective way to help bring it about?

Over the decades, Dr. Becker endeavored to guide the teaching of osteopathy in the cranial field beyond the mechanistically oriented approach that predominated in the 1950s and 60s after Sutherland's death – an approach that was largely adopted to ensure the survival of "cranial osteopathy" in an unaccepting professional environment. In his lectures and writings, Dr. Becker taught in a manner which enabled students to seek and observe those same living forces of health within the body that he had learned from. It was not until the latter part of the 1970s, with a younger generation of students, that he began to find more receptivity for integrating an understanding of the life forces at play in the delivery of health.

In his private conversations, Rollin freely spoke about his thoughts on the nature of health and healing – including the energetic and spiritual aspects as he experienced them. But for many years he mostly refrained from talking about them in his teaching. In the 1980s, Dr. Becker became more comfortable speaking in this way at courses with students. But he maintained a wariness of saying too much, in part because he found he was often misunderstood, and he found it difficult to adequately articulate these concepts. In 1988, at the age of 78, Dr. Becker retired from teaching as he was becoming disabled by vascular dementia.

Dr. Becker lived the osteopathy that he taught – it being both simple and profound. His understanding of health and healing, and his capacity to apply it for the benefit of his patients and students, were profound. Yet this great depth of knowledge and skill were always delivered in the simplest and most direct way possible. He met the needs of each person who came to him as best he could and strove to learn something more about Life from each encounter.

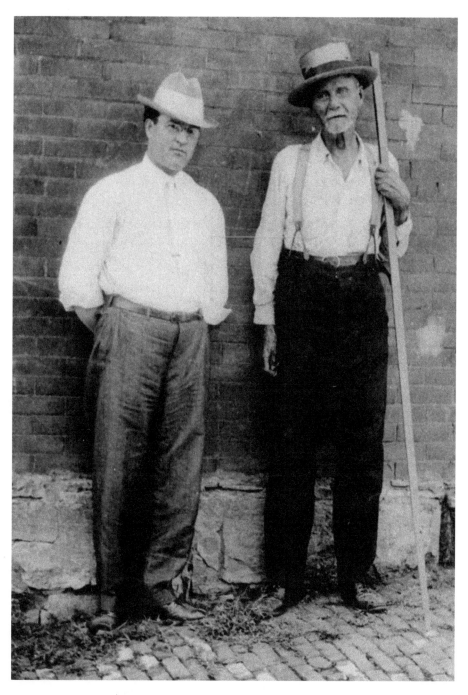

Rollin's father, Arthur D. Becker, with A. T. Still, prior to 1909.
Arthur was a faculty member at the American School of Osteopathy
in Kirksville, Missouri and later served as its dean.

Museum of Osteopathic Medicine, Kirksville, MO [cat#: 1994.1595.03].

Rollin at the Table

Mark Baker

My osteopathy teacher, Jacques Duval, would have really enjoyed this book of stories. I can hear him now. He often said it is not just what you do as an osteopath, that is, what your philosophy, knowledge, and technique are; but it is also your "osteopathic culture." For Jacques the phrase "osteopathic culture" meant where your philosophy, knowledge and technique were coming from. Who gave it to you? How had your teacher(s) received it, worked with what they had learned, and evolved? Jacques would say that the stories and personalities of our teachers; the interactions we observed and had around these older osteopaths; and, above all, the difficulties that they had to overcome, gives a different flavor and depth to what we do as osteopaths. These experiences and insights are inspiring, and at the same time these things help keep our feet on the ground. They remind us that we did not come up with this method ourselves, but we were lucky enough to meet generous people to point us in a good direction.

The first time I met Jacques was in Paris, when I went to receive a treatment in the early 1990s. We exchanged greetings and then he asked me why I was there. I replied that I heard that he had studied with Rollin Becker. Jacques suddenly looked very serious and asked, "Do you have news from Rollin? How is he?" I had to reply, "No, unfortunately, I never met him." He then took a case history and treated me.

The treatment was very enjoyable, but I had absolutely no clue what he was doing. His contact was different from anything I knew. It was very gentle, but it was like he was everywhere at the same time. Eventually, I stopped trying to figure it out as it was more pleasurable to just enjoy the experience. When the treatment was over, I asked Jacques, "Was it my fourth dorsal again?" Jacques giggled and said, "My little Mark, I stopped counting years ago."

What I had not thought to tell Jacques in the case history (patients tend to forget don't they?) was that my C3 had long ago been diagnosed as rotating right and the knob of the transverse process of C3 was always sticking out and it was always a bit tense. I probably forgot to mention it because I had had it cracked literally hundreds of times at the European School of Osteopathy by just about everybody, without a lasting change. On leaving his office Jacques warned me that "anything was possible in the next 48 hours, so don't worry about it." The next day I woke up, had a coffee, then suddenly had a feeling that someone had hit me on the back of the head with an iron bar. My headache worsened and I had to spend the day and night in bed. The day after, I awoke and had a feeling that something inside me had changed. I looked in the mirror and, honestly, my head looked different. I felt my neck, and the famous bump on C3 had gone. I felt it again, just to make sure, and it was gone and never came back. I thought back to the treatment from Jacques: He never even went near the upper cervicals. How could someone with such a gentle contact have such a powerful effect? I realized that whatever it was he was doing, I wanted to learn it from Jacques.

I spent the next 12 years studying with him. Part of the learning process took place in regular lessons, part was in treatments, and the other part was in restaurants. Jacques had a huge osteopathic culture. He had met and had experiences with so many great osteopaths and also had many stories told to him by them. I loved listening to the stories. Notably, the main character in so many of the stories was Rollin Becker. I do not think that I ever had a conversation with Jacques where at one point we did not end up talking about Rollin. Rollin was always the third person at the table. He was always with us. I never got to meet Rollin in person, but his life philosophy, palpatory approach, and treatment method have very profoundly affected me – and I am very thankful for having received this teaching.

Jacques really loved Rollin. Rollin called Jacques his spiritual brother and just loved talking about osteopathy and sharing his ideas with him. Jacques also loved talking about osteopathy and sharing his thoughts with Rollin.

One day, while at work, I received a message that Jacques was hospitalized with phlebitis. Concerned, I canceled my patients and went straight to the hospital. When I walked into his room, Jacques was lying in bed with his leg elevated and he was connected to an IV machine that would occasionally ping. He was reading a book which was the first book of Rollin's work, *Life in Motion*. With concern, I asked Jacques how he was, and Jacques looked up and said to me, "My little Mark, would you like to know what I learned about osteopathy today?" I, of course, said "Yes". He snapped the book closed and spent the next half hour telling me. Rollin was of course central in this discourse. Then he opened his book and returned to his reading, and so I knew that it was time to leave, and we bade each other goodbye. Only after leaving did I realize that I had not found out anything about his condition!

I hope you enjoy the following stories that Jacques shared with me.

Jacques Meets His Teacher

Jacques Duval, as told by Mark Baker

In 1974, Jacques attended a cranial course in Kentucky in which a senior US faculty member was lecturing. At the time, Jacques was in the early stages of his exploration of cranial osteopathy. This exploration arose out of his desire to seek an understanding and way of treating that moved beyond the "structural osteopathy" that he had practiced and taught for quite a while. At the conclusion of the lecture, Jacques asked the speaker many probing questions – wanting to dig deeper into the information that had been presented – but the speaker was unable to answer the questions and dismissed his inquiries.

In the table session that followed, Jacques was sitting with his hands on his practice partner's head with eyes closed as he concentrated on carrying out the practical session. Then, suddenly, he felt the person's mechanism begin to swing wildly from side to side in a lateral fluctuation pattern. Jacques opened his eyes and saw Rollin Becker holding onto the patient's toes and gently moving them in such a way as to create this effect. And he saw Dr. Becker was laughing with glee.

Dr. Becker then came around to the head of the table and whispered into Jacques' ear, "I know what you mean – what you are asking. If you come around to my place, I'll tell you how it works." And that is what Jacques did. For five summers he traveled from Paris, France to Dallas, Texas to stay for a month or so at the Becker's home and study with Rollin.

As for the teaching, well, it is a bit like in the film *The Matrix*, where the hero is looking everywhere for the truth. Then, at last, he finds someone who says he has the answers to all his questions, however there is a choice to make. Either you take the red pill which will reveal the truth, but you will never be the same again and you will have to dedicate your life to it; or you take the blue pill, and you will remain in blissful ignorance with a great big grin.

My understanding of the "wiggling of the toes" episode was partly just Rollin revealing his funny side. But it also seems he was saying to Jacques: "See what I can do, it is easy to mess around with a person's mechanism, but the trick is, you need to ask yourself: Where are you willing to go with this?" It was clear that Rollin wanted to share and exchange the knowledge and experience he had, and he saw Jacques' desire to learn. It was Rollin demanding presence, and Jacques chose to be fully present in this first meeting with his teacher.

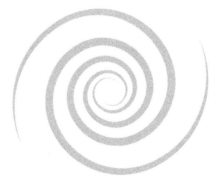

Branded His Heart

Jacques Duval, as told by Mark Baker

On his first trip to Dallas to study with Rollin,
Jacques was surprised with how things went
after they got to his office. On his first day,
Rollin told Jacques, "I am interested to see
what it is you can do," and asked him to treat
the next patient. Jacques described his reaction
as being terrified and trembling, but he sat
down and diligently gave the best cranial
treatment that he could along the lines that he
had been taught. That patient had a great deal
of tension from a chronic occipitomastoid
lesion, but by the end Jacques felt that the
occiput was floating freely.

At the end, Rollin said: "Well done, Jacques!
You went to the very depths of the superficial
tissues." Rollin then went on to say that he
wanted Jacques to "re-block" that patient's
head. Rollin told Jacques that he had taken
out every compensatory pattern the patient
had, and he should put the head back to the
way it was before because it was better then.

Understandably, Jacques' initial reaction to
Rollin's words was to feel a disappointment
in himself. But he soon saw that these words
were a wake-up call. Some gentler expression

from Rollin might not have made such an impression and Rollin was communicating to him that we do not have time to waste.

This teaching was a branding iron that indelibly marked Jacques' heart and touched him to his core. From that time on, every time he treated someone, he asked himself if he had done the job well? Had he connected his involuntary mechanism with that of his patient? Was he palpating in the way that Rollin had taught him? Were his fulcrums correctly in place? And most importantly, was his mind focused and was he fully present?

Jacques never wavered in his strong commitment to these principles – and just to make sure, he kept a picture in his treatment room of Rollin watching.

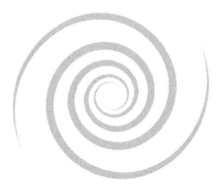

Read Between the Lines

Jacques Duval, as told by Mark Baker

During his visits to Dallas, Jacques always
stayed in the home of Dr. Becker. At the
beginning of his first visit, they were sitting
in the living room and Rollin suggested three
readings to him. The first was Chapter 10
on "The Fascia" in A.T. Still's *Philosophy of
Osteopathy*. Rollin told Jacques he should read
Still's writings three times. The first time was
to read for the words, the second time for the
understanding, and the third time to read
between the lines for the deeper meaning.

Jacques read and reread Chapter 10 a lot
more than three times. He considered it a
cornerstone of Rollin's teaching – Jacques felt
that it fueled his embryological approach,
served as a definition of the "involuntary," and
was the basis of his diagnosis and treatment
method. The contents of this chapter came
up in Jacques' conversations and lectures
all the time. Jacques recommended that all
osteopaths read it three times and draw their
own conclusions

Next, Rollin asked Jacques if he knew
of the French priest, Pierre Teilhard de
Chardin? Jacques was somewhat embarrassed

to admit that he did not know of this fellow Frenchman. Rollin, a little puzzled, told Jacques that it would be most beneficial for him to get up to date on this man. De Chardin was a catholic priest who was a deep thinker. However, his views and way of explaining the universe and the evolution of consciousness was distinctly different from his church's orthodoxy, which sometimes got him into a lot of trouble. I know that Jacques took Rollin's advice and read de Chardin, but I do not know what he made of his writings. De Chardin's work is difficult to encapsulate into a simple set of theories. My own sense is that what he is describing in his own words is what we would call the involuntary, and that his ideas helped Rollin in his own understanding and explanations.

Lastly, he recommended that Jacques read the books of Walter Russell. When speaking of Walter Russell, Jacques would tell me that Russell deeply influenced Rollin's understanding of stillness. Rollin used a double spiral diagram, which comes up a lot in Russell's work, to explain life in motion with its fulcrum in stillness.

This Extraordinary Calm

Jacques Duval, as told by Mark Baker

When Jacques came from Paris to study with Rollin in Dallas, he could not have imagined what Rollin's office would be like. He knew Rollin to be a highly skilled and highly respected osteopathic physician, and so he was not expecting to see Rollin's office set between a burger place, with a large plywood cowboy on a horse in the window to the right, and what appeared to be some sort of adult erotic shop on the left. Entering Rollin's office, Jacques noted the not-very-pleasing wood paneling on the walls with jokes plastered all over the waiting room. These visual effects were somewhat jarring to him, but then there was the issue of the noise.

Because there was no real sound buffer between the treatment room and the waiting room, Rollin had obtained the noisiest air conditioner that he could find so that patients in the waiting room could not hear what was going on in the treatment room. The fan made a terrible clanking sound that Jacques described as producing a horrendous amount of noise. He would say you could not even hear yourself think.

And yet, despite this menagerie of noise and distraction, Jacques experienced this extraordinary calm feeling in the room that Rollin seemed to generate. With Rollin present, there was an amazing stillness in the room – unaffected by the surroundings. This was another important lesson for Jacques. Whenever he told this story it was obvious the reverence Jacques had for the power of presence that was Rollin, and he would always end by saying: "We must emulate this."

Not Too Seriously

Jacques Duval, as told by Mark Baker

Another lesson Jacques took away from his
time in Rollin's office was the idea of not taking
oneself too seriously. He saw that Rollin did
not take himself that seriously. Clearly, Rollin
took his work very seriously, but he did not take
himself that seriously. He never made himself out
to be better than anyone else or to be like a guru.
His teachings were, from what I heard and read,
never direct – he would not say that this means
that. His teachings were always very open and
something to be pondered about for a long time.

There was one poster in Rollin's waiting room
that was quite large, and written in big letters
it said: For any complaints about the service on
these premises please fill in the box below. The
box was of course the size of a small postage
stamp. From this joke, we can imagine that
Rollin actively encouraged patients not to take
themselves too seriously either.

Early Guidance

Rachel Brooks

I first met Dr. Becker in 1975, just a week before I entered medical school; and much of the time that I got to spend with him in the following years was long before I was a fully formed practitioner. Some of the wisdom he imparted to me had an immediate impact, while other parts of it took years and years to unfold their meaning. There were a couple of things he told me early on that made a big difference in my life from the start and continue to guide me almost 50 years later. The two things I want to share are distinct, but I find them also inter-related.

Dr. Becker once said that one reason to not take the credit when a patient gets better is because if you do, you also then have to take the blame when the patient does not get better. This struck me as a good idea. With this in mind, from the start of my practice life, whenever a patient expressed their gratitude and praise to me for resolving their problem, I replied by saying something along these lines: "Osteopathy is a powerful and wonderful approach, and I am grateful it was able to help you."

Of course, being human, it does feel really good to receive patients' praise for all the good, and sometimes remarkably good, results achieved; but it also then can feel demoralizing to experience the sometimes-puzzling lack of a positive outcome. To this day, whenever I speak those words of shifting the praise away from myself and towards osteopathy, I think of what Dr. Becker said. And I also try to remember what he said when the disappointments inevitably happen as well.

This guidance from Dr. Becker helps me as I approach my day-to-day work – I strive to do the best I can for each patient, and I hope it will be of help to them. This is where the advice of "not taking the credit" connects to the second piece of guidance I want to share, that of "not being attached to the outcome."

Dr. Becker was really clear about the importance of not being attached to the outcome of our treatments. He would say that our job is to give the best treatment we can, and what the patient or patient's mechanism does with it is up to them. We do all we can to marshal the patient's resources and remove all the obstacles we can, but the outcome may or may not be what we or the patient might hope for.

In other discussions around this subject, Dr. Becker encouraged me to see that we cannot know what the arc of that person's life journey is. My understanding of what he was saying is that we might assume the patient has arrived on our doorstep to be relieved of their suffering, but we cannot know that. We do not know what role we will be playing in their lives. Once again, our job is to be present for them and give the best care that we can.

The guidance Dr. Becker gave to me while I was a student and young practitioner was precious. While I would, not surprisingly, need to absorb these lessons over and over again, they have given me a treasured framework in which to grow as a practitioner and person.

Not Strictly Mechanical

Thomas Thrall

My first exposure to osteopathy came in 1975, when I was in my sophomore year of medical school. Dr. Becker had come to meet with a small group of allopathic medical students who were all connected with a spiritual community. In that gathering he gave an informal presentation of his work and the basic principles of osteopathy.

Even though none of us had yet been taught to perceive the movement of the primary respiratory mechanism, Dr. Becker had us get to the tables. He then instructed us to place our hands under the patient's head, relax, open our minds, and simply see if something happened.

As we began this exercise, Dr. Becker stepped over to the far corner of the room, lit his pipe, and sat quietly. About five minutes into the session, I did think that I was beginning to feel "something happening," although I had no idea if it was what I was supposed to feel or not. I looked up to see if I might catch Dr. Becker's attention for a moment to ask him about it and found that he was already staring right at me! He then said clearly and directly to me, "There, did you feel that?"

For me, it was remarkable that at the very start of my osteopathic life, I was able to have this experience. Dr. Becker's ability to sense the change from across the room like that was also meaningful. It led me to understand right away that this approach to healing was not strictly mechanical.

Focus on Anatomy

Richard Holding

Rollin was my key inspiration – he made me want to be a true osteopath. Before meeting him, I believe I was what I might call a musculoskeletal practitioner. On my first course with Rollin in 1975, I sat listening to him and he had this amazing vision of this beautiful way to work – and I knew that is what I wanted to do.

One of the first things Rollin did with me was to take me back to anatomy. In those years when he came to England to teach, he would spend time in my home in Herefordshire. After dinner, with either whiskey or wine in hand, the portable treatment table would go up and we would explore osteopathy. In was then that he focused me on anatomy and introduced me to the Bassett slides. The Bassett Collection included 1,547 stereoscopic images allowing one to see the anatomy in three dimensions which made spatial awareness in the tissues much easier to visualize.

After he left, I bought a set of the Bassett slides so I could work with my patients and look up the anatomy. That really developed precision for me in practice, and I still consult them sometimes. Bringing anatomy to life was really important to me – it is that care and precision and the development of visualization that I think is fundamental to my being an osteopath.

Carefully Watching

Richard Holding

On one of his teaching trips to England, Rollin spent a day in my office seeing patients with me during one of his stays at my house. On that day, every time I closed my eyes, he gave me a kick under the table. He told me that if you close your eyes, it is too easy to "windshield wipe," as he called it. If you go inside and concentrate, he said it is too easy to go on autopilot doing various things and have your treatments stay superficial. If you have your eyes open and you are paying attention, applying anatomical-physiological visualization to what is happening under your hands, and projecting awareness into areas that you cannot see, you can go more deeply. That is what we were doing when we were working together.

I had been thinking that if you close your eyes, you can concentrate more, but I had bruises on my legs in learning otherwise from Rollin! He was keenly observing, looking, and very carefully watching while treating. It has taken me many years to see even vaguely what he saw.

The other thing that came up when we were working with this was what he called the "Twin Threaded Screw" approach. Apparently there existed a kind of screw you could put into a wall that had another part that you could put in and it could be screwed back out. (It seems, what Rollin was calling a twin threaded screw, would now be called a *threaded anchor with screw.*) No one else I have talked to about this heard him use this term, but it was an analogy he shared with me. When he was working, he would sit using what he called his "listening posts," which were his hands, and he described projecting down into the tissue using anatomical-physiological visualization to identify what was going on under his hands. He then shared how he would stay there with one part of his awareness while he also would wind back out to be aware of the universality of the person.

How Is It Functioning?

Nicholas Handoll

There were a couple statements Dr. Becker made at different times that helped to impress upon me the understanding that how the body is functioning is at the core of osteopathic diagnosis and treatment.

In a course with Dr. Becker, he told us that when seeing a patient for the first time, we should take a proper case history, make all the appropriate clinical examinations, order all the tests and imaging we need, consider all the differential diagnoses, and finally come to the diagnosis of what is wrong. Then we should parcel it all up inside a box, tie a ribbon around it, and for the time of the treatment push it to one side and ask the Mechanism what it wants.

As a relative beginner in the field of cranial osteopathy this was a simple and clear guidance about the central importance of function. Knowledge of anatomy, physiology, and clinical diagnosis is crucial, but in practicing osteopathy we should always remember that the key question is ultimately: How is it functioning?

In another course, Dr. Becker had finished the morning session with talk about the central nervous system. He concluded the discussion by saying that we would talk about the pineal gland after lunch, and he asked us to consider the pineal gland over lunch. Eager students that we were, we pretty much forgot about lunch and spent our time reviewing the anatomy and physiology of the gland: where it was located, what it secreted, what role it played in the body…. After lunch we shared all the information that we had gathered with Dr. Becker, who listened carefully. "That's fascinating," he said, "but how does it move?"

Fluid Drive

Maxwell Fraval

Dr. Rollin Becker was part of the Sutherland Cranial Teaching
Foundation faculty that had come to teach a cranial course in the UK
around 1980. At the end of the course, Dr. Becker was the faculty
member to "check my head" to make sure I wasn't leaving the course
with any new strains. As I lay on the table, he just placed his hands
under my occiput and sat, and it seemed to me he just observed the
mechanism for what seemed like a long time (but was maybe only five
minutes). And then he slipped a hand down to my left fifth rib at the
costovertebral articulation.

I hadn't said anything to Dr. Becker about this, but that rib had been
a source of considerable trouble for five years. A poorly applied high
velocity technique had left me with episodic incapacitating spasm that
various osteopathic treatments had not been able to resolve.

Dr. Becker sat there with a slight lift on the rib for a few minutes. As he
released his contact he said: "The fluid is going all the way down now."
This experience was hugely important to me. For the next five years in
my practice, I treated using fluid drive most of the time. That experience
of Dr. Becker releasing that recalcitrant rib let me understand that it
really was possible to learn from inside what was needed. The reality of
listening, following, and being a witness to the healing forces within the
patient sank deeply into my consciousness.

Sick Tissues

David Douglas-Mort

Rollin came over to teach in the UK in the mid-1970s, and my wife, Rowan, and I were lucky enough to be allocated to Rollin's tutor group on the third day. It was the first Sutherland Cranial Teaching Foundation course we had attended. We knew very little of the cranial concept and by the third day our mechanisms had crashed.

Rollin started treating Rowan to get her through the course, and I asked if I could palpate whilst he treated her. He agreed and I palpated her chest whilst feeling what I was typically feeling at that time in my first cranial course, which was nothing. I was sitting there feeling just her clothing and musculature when he looked up at me, and instantly I could "see" my whole ventricular system highlighted in bright white sparkling light. It did not come through my hands. It was as though part of me was sitting inside my head as this vision of the ventricles appeared in me. I did not know what had happened, but it certainly intrigued me. How did he do that?

This extraordinary experience completely wiped out any thoughts or feelings I had at the time. But when Rollin had resurrected Rowan's mechanism after about 10 minutes, I managed to ask him what I could do in treatment to help Rowan's mechanism.

Rollin (who I later learned could be a man of few words) responded:

"CV4............, twice a week................................, for a year."

It was only years later I came to realize he was informing me of his "sick tissues make poor changes" rule. Rowan's mechanism was sick and the way to facilitate it to move to health, was to apply CV4 many times over as the first step. As tissue health returned and the potency became manifest, then her mechanism would change for the better.

It worked out just as Rollin predicted!

Probably a Witch

Caroline Tosh

I was very lucky to have had Dr. Becker as my table tutor, twice, on his trips to the UK. The second time this occurred was when I was taking my third basic cranial course. By this time, I had a bit of clinical experience with the work, and in that course I was able to perceive more. During the table session on the CV4, the instruction was given to wait, and to watch for where the fluid return comes from.

I was watching and waiting and eventually felt some fluid movement coming from the patient's pelvis with a sort of wave coming up the core and on up into the head. After I described this to Dr. Becker, a student sitting nearby commented: "I never felt anything like that before." Dr. Becker turned to the student and said, "Well, she has long fingers. She's probably a witch. Witches have long fingers you know…." It was a funny thing to say, but at the time it felt like his way of acknowledging that what I was feeling was real – that I might have a real affinity for this work. In my various encounters with Dr. Becker, he was very validating and supportive, which was a great gift to me as a young developing practitioner.

Works So Differently

Caroline Tosh

I once commented to Dr. Becker how he seemed to work so differently from Anne Wales (as they were both close students of Dr. Sutherland). I told him how it seemed to me that Anne worked so specifically with the fluid-tissue motion and in his approach to treatment, one seemed to be waiting for the Tide to show you where to go. He did not really respond to my depictions of their differences, he only said: "But Anne has the ability to sense everything that's happening in the body all the time." In this interchange I heard the great respect he had for Anne, and the lesson I took from it was his belief that we each have our own strengths and way of doing things in this work. This helped me to feel more at ease with how I worked – understanding that I did not have to work like my teachers in order to be an accomplished practitioner in my own right.

Getting the Treatment Going

Thomas Thrall

One time, when a small group of us were meeting with Dr. Becker, he talked about how to connect with a patient. He began with the basics of getting your hands in place and being relaxed and in balance. Then he talked about being aware of the inner physician – both your own and the patient's. He made the point that it is this awareness of the inner physician in this way that starts a conversation that unfolds into the treatment. He said that it is not what you do with your hands that gets a treatment going.

Later in that discussion he addressed a situation that sometimes arises in the treatment process, wherein the patient's mechanism seems to be just wandering about. It does not begin to engage or come into focus as you would expect. In this situation, he told us to get very grounded, feeling a line of connection "all the way down to the center of the earth," and then firmly instruct the patient's mechanism to "get to work."

As a young physician, this lesson from Dr. Becker made a strong impression on me about the role and power of our awareness and intentions. Over the years, when I encountered a patient's wandering mechanism, I followed his advice and told it to "get to work," and it did – it always worked.

Faith in the Mechanism

Rachel Brooks

At the end of a 40-hour Sutherland Cranial Teaching Foundation course in 1988, there was a participant who had not been able to perceive the motion of the primary respiratory mechanism at all. It was unusual at the end of such a course to have someone who had no sense of having felt the motion. This woman had a history of many accidents, and her own mechanism was quite locked-up, which was probably what was making it hard for her to perceive with her hands. This situation was brought to Dr. Becker's attention while I happened to be standing beside him. As we walked to the table where she was, I recall thinking, as a fairly new faculty person, about what I would tell her if it were me giving her advice. I thought I would tell her not to worry about her difficulty perceiving and recommend that she go home and get some treatment for her own compressed mechanism, then she would be able to develop this palpatory skill.

Dr. Becker, however, gave her some distinctly different advice. He suggested she go home to her practice, have a clock positioned where she could see it, put her hands on the area of the patient that she thought needed help, and then sit there attentively for seven minutes. He told her that something useful for the patient's problem would most likely take place in that timeframe. Hearing this, I was struck by his complete faith in the patient's mechanism to respond to such a basic approach of presence and intention.

Since then, I have often shared this story with students and young practitioners who are doubting their own skills and capacity to do this work. For me the powerful lesson was that it is far more important that we have faith in the mechanism than that we have faith in ourselves.

It's Alive!

Nicholas Handoll

One of the things that resonated with me in Dr. Becker's lectures helped me in my own search for understanding in osteopathy. He talked about the body being alive. With passion, he would say again and again: It is *alive*; it is a *living* body! He kept emphasizing this and it really did resonate – leading me to the importance of understanding exactly what a *living* organism is.

These words of Dr. Becker led me to search for a definition of what being alive meant. I came to see that a living organism is a system that constantly renews, regenerates, and reforms itself in order to remain alive and healthy. "Constantly" is the key word here.

It is not renewing, regenerating and reforming because of disease, injury or infirmity. It renews, regenerates and reforms because it is alive! It is what living systems do. This is why and how osteopathy works. We are not fixing the body–it is *renewing, regenerating,* and *reforming* anyway. We are removing the factors that are preventing it from doing so, or as Dr. Becker would say, preventing it from "expressing health." The approach works because: it is *alive*!

It has even led me to question one of the long-held and oft-quoted tenets within osteopathic practice – the word "heal." What is healing? Are we really healers? Does the body heal itself? Firstly, it begs the question: Healing from what? Disease? Do osteopaths treat "disease"?

Secondly, while the osteopath helps a patient to recover by removing the factors which are compromising health, the body will naturally concentrate its activity where it is specially needed, but is the body doing anything different from what it does normally in health by virtue of being alive? It is still renewing, regenerating, and reforming – in other words, it is being a "living" organism. Therefore, is this response "healing" or is it freeing the delivery of the constant dynamic expression of life?

Rhythmic Balanced Interchange

Caroline Penn

One phrase I heard Dr. Becker talk about in a lecture had a big impact on me and sparked an important development in my work. The phrase, "rhythmic balanced interchange," helped me put words to what I had been feeling with my patients, and it was like I had been waiting years for someone to say them.

"Rhythmic balanced interchange" resonated with the daily experience I had been having with every patient. Whenever I had felt I was in the right place, that is what was happening, but I had not had any words for it. This was a really significant lesson. That phrase served to validate my perceptions and it invited me to learn more.

Instead of wondering if what I was doing in a treatment was "right," I now knew that this was an experience of human function under my hands that I could trust. In essence, if I was in that place, it was OK to just "be" there. It gave me permission to stay with that which was important – to understand that I could ignore any temptation to follow things. It was hugely significant because it allowed me to give myself permission to stay in the process that was happening in that spot. And it has continued to serve me and my patients well ever since.

The Stillness

Rachel Brooks

I believe it was in 1979, during one of our informal
times together, Rollin and I were sitting in the
living room chatting, and he asked me if I was able
to feel the tidal motion of the primary respiratory
mechanism (PRM). At the time, it was still quite
early in the development of my palpatory skills, but
I had in fact just gotten to the point where I could
fairly reliably feel the rhythmic movement. And so,
with just a hint of pride, I told him that, yes, I could
now feel it. He replied, "Well, you know it's not the
motion that is important." Actually, no, I didn't know
that – the PRM motion seemed to be at the very core
of "cranial osteopathy" teaching. For a moment I felt
a bit deflated having put a lot of effort into feeling the
motion. And then Dr. Becker simply said, "It is the
Stillness that is important."

This one brief statement launched me into a
decades-long practice of finding for myself that deep
connection to Stillness that was so clearly manifest
in him. Dr. Becker's ability to sit in Stillness while
treating was profound and inspiring.

After hearing Dr. Becker's guidance about Stillness, I
embarked on my path of discovery working to become
more still – more attuned to Stillness – particularly
in my meditation practice. My visits with Dr. Becker

happened on an irregular basis, so a year or more could pass and then I would have the opportunity to see him again. The first time I was going to see him after his "Stillness" comment to me, I felt I had made some progress – that I could attune to Stillness some. But when I got in Rollin's presence while he was treating, I experienced the magnitude of this state of Stillness that was so very much more than I had encountered on my own. Observing this, I said to myself, "Oh, he means being *really* still."

So, I returned home and carried on with my practice of attending to Stillness, and over time, had a sense of having made more progress; then I'd have a chance to be with Dr. Becker again; and once more was struck by the profound manifestation of Stillness in his presence. In response, I said to myself, "Oh, he means being *really, really* still." And that is how it went for every encounter I had with Rollin after that. I would always come away thinking, "Oh, he means being *really, really, really* still." Rollin pointing me toward the experience of Stillness changed my life.

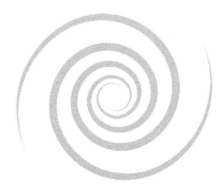

Infinite Possibilities

Richard Holding

After a day of his teaching at a course in London, Rollin and I went back to my hotel room to treat my wife, Karen. Before treating, he read aloud a passage from one of his favorite authors, Loren Eiseley, a naturalist and popular science writer. Rollin then proceeded to illuminate the Stillness in the whole of Karen. In this practical way, Rollin was able to introduce me to the infinite possibilities inherent in Stillness; that Stillness both goes back in time and into the future and is, at the same time, radically present. This is the passage that he read to us:

> "Imagine for a moment, that you have drunk from a magician's goblet. Reverse the irreversible stream of time. Go down the dark stairwell out of which the race has ascended. Find yourself at last on the bottommost steps of time, slipping, sliding, and wallowing by scale and fin down into the muck and ooze out of which you arose. Pass by grunts and hissings below the last tree ferns. Eyeless and earless, float in the primal waters, sense sunlight you cannot see and stretch absorbing tentacles towards vague tastes that float in water. Still, in your formless shiftings, the you remains: the sliding particles, the juices, the transformations are working in an exquisitely patterned rhythm which has no other purpose than your preservation – you, the entity, the amoeboid being whose substance contains the unfathomable future. Even so does every man come upwards from the waters of his birth."
>
> (From *The Immense Journey* by Loren Eiseley.)

For Rollin this was an archetypal description for the descent into Stillness.

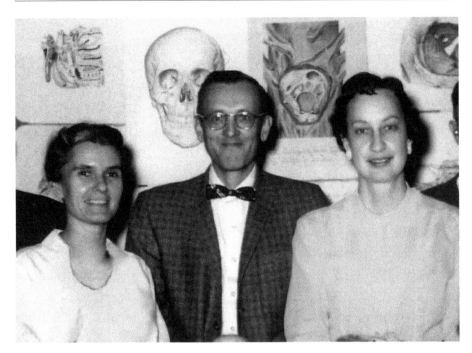

Faculty at a "Refresher Course" in Los Angeles, 1959. Left to Right: Viola Frymann, Rollin Becker, Edna Lay. Dr. Becker is holding a teaching skull in his hands that is not shown in this cropped photo.

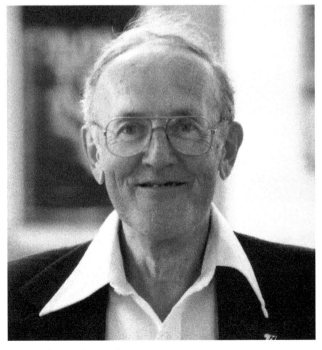

Dr. Becker in the mid-1980s.

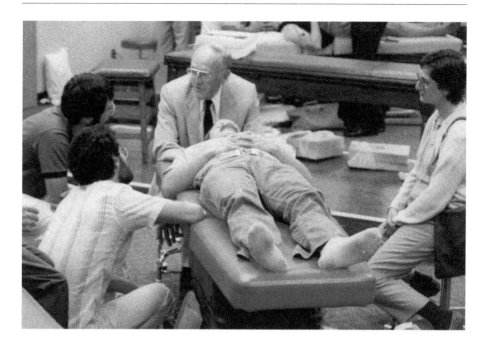

Dr. Becker teaching at an SCTF course in Fort Worth, Texas, 1984.
Pictured at right is Rachel Brooks and at the bottom is Mark Rosen,
other students unidentified. Photos by Donald Becker, MD.

Top photo: Museum of Osteopathic Medicine, Kirksville, MO [cat#: 2011.01.208].

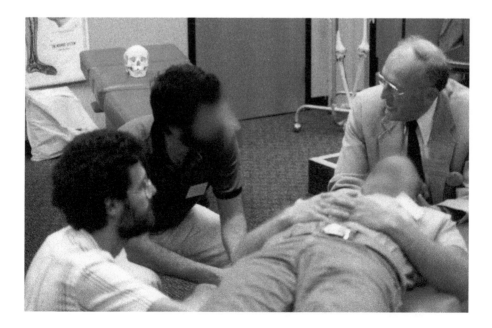

One Whole Tone

Caroline Tosh

Sometime in the early 1980s, between my second and third cranial course, I had a vivid, but strange and puzzling experience. My office at the time had a mulberry tree in the yard outside the window, and whilst I was treating, I used to mentally "be" the mulberry tree as a way to anchor my attention. One day during a treatment, this patient became still, and then even more still and more still. He became so still that he appeared to be pixelating – like in a cartoon where the substance starts to break into little pieces and very slowly change, come apart, and then come back together. When things had fully come back together, I was aware of a particular feeling in which I felt that there was one whole tone in the patient.

I did not understand this experience at the time, and asked my various teachers in the UK if they had ever had an experience like that – where the patient goes so still that you feel there is just one whole tone in the patient? No one said that they had – so I just kept on working and wondering, and it did not happen again. Then at my third basic course, I decided to ask Dr. Becker, who had come as the guest faculty. I said to him: "Dr. Becker, I had this very weird experience with a patient where he went so very still, he just became little pieces that were moving, spreading, and coming back together again; and when the patient came back together, they were more homogenous and there was one whole tone. Do you think that when the patient is really, really still there is just one homogenous tone – is this possible?"

In response, Dr. Becker just smiled and said, "Yep." That is all he said, but it was so positive a reply it let me know that I was not crazy and maybe I was on the right track. I did not have any other patient go disappearing under my hands like that for many years until I learned to go there more deliberately, understanding it to be a point of dynamic stillness. I just blundered into it that first time, but I am grateful I did.

That's Interesting

Rachel Brooks

In our conversations, Rollin would talk about Will Sutherland's use of the phrase "Why not?" It was a comment Will often made when replying to one of his students after they had shared with him some idea or conclusion they had come to about an aspect of the cranial concept or some notion about the larger nature of things.

While "why not?" could be interpreted as an affirmative response – indicating that the idea presented had merit – Rollin understood it could be interpreted otherwise. He described Will's meaning to be more like: Maybe you are getting on to something and maybe not; either way you might want to keep digging in order to deepen and clarify your understanding.

My observation was that Rollin had his own way of replying when a student presented some idea or interpretation that he thought was not entirely on track; was incomplete; or was about something that was fundamentally unknowable. In these instances, I often heard him say "That's interesting" or "That's very interesting"; or he had a way of shrugging his shoulders that also implied: Maybe that's true, maybe that's not, or maybe we just can't know. In my experience, if you had landed on some truth that he could affirm – he might say "yep" and leave it at that; or he might simply give a small nod of his head and with an inner smile on his face, quietly say, "that's right."

Hit a Wall

Anthony Norrie

In 1988, I attended my first Sutherland Cranial Teaching Foundation Basic Course in the US and had wanted to spend some time with Rollin Becker to see and experience what it was that made him a legend. However, I did not get any time with him at the tables and was feeling disappointed by not having had that opportunity. Then, towards the end of the course, I saw an elderly couple enter the room. It became clear they were there for the woman to be treated by Dr. Becker. Being young and brash I thought that this was my opportunity to see what he did that was so special.

As the woman lay down on the table and Dr. Becker began the treatment, I started off across the room so I could be close to them and observe the treatment. But as I was striding towards Dr. Becker, I literally bounced off an invisible wall. I actually tried to get through this barrier three times, but each time I could not penetrate the unseen field.

I was dumbfounded by this unusual circumstance, but I did finally realize that there was no possibility of getting past this wall. I did not experience this as an active exclusion; at the time, I was simply perplexed as to what I had just experienced.

It took many years before I began to understand what had happened, and this was a two-fold journey. One aspect of this journey was developing my perceptual awareness and experience of stillness. An important part of that lesson from Dr. Becker came during a presentation by Dr. Brooks. She had recently been to visit him after he had become disabled, and I was dumbstruck by my experience of the entire room going into a very deep still point as soon as she put her photo of the great man on the screen. The other aspect, conjoined with the first, was my personal journey of resolving that which keeps me apart from stillness.

What I understand now is that in my enthusiasm for an experience, I did not know that I could not be a part of something that I was not invited into. Also, because of all that I was carrying in my own being that kept me from being conscious of stillness, this meant that there was no possible physical way that I could have entered the therapeutic cocoon that Dr. Becker had created for this person.

Sometimes you need to be hit with a baseball bat, or an invisible field, to set you on a path of discovery.

The Ethereal Organ

Caroline Penn

In a 1988 lecture at a Sutherland Cranial Teaching Foundation course in England, Dr. Becker gave a lecture in which he offered us information about the movement of the central nervous system and a picture of how the fluid moved around and through the cranium. He made a particular point about the importance of the cerebrospinal fluid (CSF) moving through the cribriform plate in relation to the olfactory bulbs.

Dr. Becker could not have guessed that someone in the audience was missing one of their olfactory bulbs. However, I was missing one, and I felt some distress as he carried on in his lecture about the valuable role those bulbs played. Eleven years earlier I had been struck by a car and sustained a head injury with a fracture through the roof of the orbit extending into the cribriform plate. During a surgical procedure to repair the torn membrane that was allowing a CSF leak, one of the olfactory bulbs was removed (I subsequently learned that the membrane problem most likely would have healed on its own without surgery.).

Because of the distress I felt from his lecture, I caught up with Dr. Becker afterwards and asked him what it meant if one was missing? I asked whether I should be worried that I had only one? He immediately reassured me by saying I needn't worry because "the ethereal olfactory bulb is still there."

Reflecting back now on that interaction with Dr. Becker about my olfactory bulb, I am particularly struck with this realization: Although I've experienced some extremes of sensory olfactory function over the years, as I look back over the 40 years since that accident, I can report that my olfaction has actually improved.

Acknowledging the Shock

Caroline Penn

In his writings, Dr. Becker gives an account of a man who had a peripheral injury in his leg, and he describes the work that was accomplished by acknowledging the shock at the level of the spinal cord. When I read this long ago, it had a profound impact on me; it hit me right between the eyes and it is something I have carried through my work for all these years.

These days when I am working with people, I spend a good deal of time being aware of how their body is processing shock. I notice whether they are able to process shock well, not so well, or barely at all; and I notice all the different nuances of shock. Rollin really opened up that internal dialogue for me.

Dr. Becker's approach also invited me to think about the shock from my own road traffic accident, and as a result, the effects from that old trauma transformed into a new experience for me. As is often the case after head injury, I had total anosmia. This was true for eight years, even though I still had one olfactory bulb intact. Rollin's words extended an invitation for me to look at that shock in a different way – to go right to the depth of it, acknowledging the oneness of everything and experiencing the shock.

When my sense of smell did return it was super-sensitive. My own interpretation of the situation (reinforced by my study of the HANDLE method) is that right after the accident, my sense of smell was so heightened and overwhelming that my body's natural stress response was to shut the system down completely. Given this, it would not be surprising that a part of releasing the shock was to go through a phase of hypersensitive olfaction.

So many insights I have had about myself and my patients go back to what Rollin was saying about how it is that we can acknowledge and treat the shock that resides in our bodies.

Editor's note: HANDLE is designed to enhance neurological systems that are causing learning or life difficulties. See https://handle.org

How Our Palpation Works

R. Paul Lee

During a break at my first basic cranial course, Dr. Becker and I were the last two remaining at the lunch table. Before returning to the classroom, he told me to observe the brain, as it emits sensory information from the somatosensory cortex just as the ears emit sound waves and the eyes emit light. I was a relative youngster in osteopathy at the time and did not know what to make of this unusual statement made without context, but I did understand that this was a simple gesture of sharing his insights. I never have been quite sure I understood what he was describing, but I have always appreciated that moment of contact with this respected osteopathic elder.

Curiously, just recently I came across a few lines in his book that expressed what he had told me. For a piece I am writing, I had been searching for a totally different quote of Dr. Becker's and decided that a good way to find it was to reread *Life in Motion* and *The Stillness of Life*. I was having fun reading through those books again and came across this quotation: "The art and science of palpation can be enhanced in both quantity and quality by learning to consciously project the sense of touch from the sensory area of the brain through to the hands by way of the proprioceptive neural pathways as well as the tactile endings, rather than passively waiting for sensory input to be transmitted from the hands to the sensory centers in the brain." (*Life in Motion*, p.56)

That is the essence of what Dr. Becker told me back in the 1980s before I knew what to make of it. Reading that passage in the book, I felt gratified that I had come to the same realization over the course of my practice life. This is how I teach people to feel nuclei in the brain, for instance. I have long pondered the question, how does our palpation work? Over the years, I have had various revelations that informed my own thinking and experience. In 2017, I got my ideas down in an article for The Cranial Letter titled, "Palpation: Electric or magnetic?" I do not know if Dr. Becker would agree with everything I wrote, but having just read his thoughts on the matter, I'm pretty sure he would appreciate the line of thought.

Life Force and the Tree

Richard Holding

On one of Rollin's visits, I had an important experience that took me quite a long time to appreciate the depth of its meaning for me. On Rollin's various trips to the UK to teach in the 1970s, he would come and stay for a time at my house in the countryside, which had a beautiful garden on seven acres of land. On the property was this wonderful 150-year-old copper beech tree that he loved going to look at.

During that particular visit, probably in 1979, he read to me the paper he had recently written entitled, "Motion: The Key to Diagnosis and Treatment" (see *Life in Motion*). In that paper he introduced his concept of the long tide, and after the reading Rollin took me out to the garden. He first had me touch a young developing tree and asked, "What do you feel?" I responded that I felt a lightness in the tree. Then we both got our hands on the beech tree and I could feel this incredible powerful surging. We spent some time there with Rollin showing me the frequency of the long tide in the tree.

While I still had my hands on the beech tree, Rollin walked away and, turning to the young tree, he made a comment that I might want to take that tree down just to make space. Then he turned back to me and said, "You should do the same to the big tree," and I was hit by the palpatory experience of the tree's emphatic response. I had the feeling of it responding with a clear feeling of "no chance;" the tree did not think this was a good idea.

At the time I was most taken with the manifestation of life and power in that tree – the power of that tree being fully present. But, gradually, over some years that experience led me to think about the effect negative thoughts and energies have on people. I believe Rollin's lesson to me went beyond a demonstration about the long tide. Over time, I have come to see it as a demonstration that there are a lot of life experiences which are limiting us and there are life experiences which are enhancing. If one is in a state of dysfunction or disunity, then it is very hard to discriminate between those, and it allows these negative influences to have a much more fundamental discordant effect on the body. That was a great lesson for me.

This has led me to looking at long-term difficult stress patterns in our patient's physiology through the prism of trauma where these negative influences leave trauma imprints in the tissues, which alter their integration with the Whole.

The Macrocosm Within Us

Richard Holding

During Rollin's visits he would talk about the
scientist-philosopher Walter Russell's influence
on Will Sutherland and himself. He pointed out
that it was from Russell's *The Divine Iliad* that
we have the language of the cranial approach.
For me, it is historically very important that
we realize that Reciprocal Tension, the Light,
Stillness, the Fulcrum, etc. are all fundamental
principles of the Universe (the macrocosm) that
are within us as well (the microcosm).

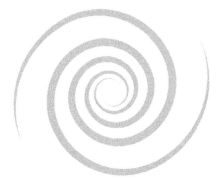

Master Fulcrum

Richard Holding

In the 1970s when Rollin was coming to teach in England and we spent time together, during our discussions he often used the term "master fulcrum." At times I have been asked whether the master fulcrum and Sutherland's Fulcrum are the same thing? In answer I can only say that Rollin seemed to use the terms interchangeably. My understanding is that before some of Dr. Sutherland's faculty gave this fulcrum point their teacher's name, it was called the master fulcrum.

My own reflection now is that Rollin might have continued using the terminology of the master fulcrum as a way of maintaining a more expansive view of its function. It seems to me that Sutherland's Fulcrum came to be described in more anatomical and mechanical ways – maybe feeling a need to move away from the controversy that existed (and still exists) in the medical world in relation to "energy" medicine. Personally, I see the Master Fulcrum encompassing the "Whole" of the being, including the Subtle Bodies.

Read Quantum Mechanics

Nicholas Handoll

During one of the courses that Dr. Becker taught at the British School of Osteopathy in the 1970s, I caught up with him between lectures and asked a question: What do you think is the driving force of this mechanism? At the time the lecturers had been talking of a physical movement driven by the cerebrospinal fluid, but I was beginning to experience that this movement could be a response to something external. So, I asked him what was making it move? I said that I thought it could be something coming from outside the body. Dr. Becker replied, "Read quantum mechanics," and walked off.

I didn't know at the time that he was known as a man of few words and that his short reply was typical in such a setting. I had suspected he was just trying to get rid of the young guy asking annoying questions. Whatever Dr. Becker's intention was, spurred by his words, the study of quantum mechanics became a lifetime endeavor for me. Eventually this study led me to a viewpoint that deeply informed my osteopathic approach and was the motivation for writing *The Anatomy of Potency* and for developing the course Energy Osteopathy.

My research led me to re-evaluate osteopathy. It has honed my understanding of what Dr. Still was trying to say. It has made me re-evaluate what is real – what is reality. What really is this world, the environment in which we live? I know now it is not what we commonly think. The more I delved into quantum reality the more it made sense and prompted me to question my experience and view of existence – and it clarified Still's philosophy.

It has shown me that we humans are just a miniscule microcosm of the greater environment in which we exist. This vision of humanity somehow resonates with Rollin's statement that frequently slipped into his lectures telling us we needed to: "Get your big fat egos out of the way."

I believe that Dr. Sutherland had experiences and insights into this greater understanding of the primary respiratory mechanism (PRM), but in his lifetime, he did not feel free to speak of this aspect within the profession. So, he felt he could only describe the PRM for us as a mechanical/physiological phenomenon. Quantum mechanics leads me to see the PRM as being the image in the sensorium of one living human being (the practitioner) in relation or in response to another living human being within the overwhelming energy and power of our cosmic environment.

Stand on Their Shoulders

Rachel Brooks

Dr. Becker held a strong belief that it was a student's right (and maybe responsibility) to "stand on the shoulders" of their teacher. He believed that students could gain what knowledge and skills that they could from their teachers and then go on to develop their own, hopefully greater, understanding.

Connected with this idea was his belief that what you had taken into yourself from your mentors became yours. If you study his lectures and writings, you will see that he rarely names the source of the information and ideas he is presenting. Rollin certainly had the most profound respect and gratitude for what he had received from the lineage of Drs. Still and Sutherland, but he believed the reality was that he had imbibed and digested the knowledge to the best of his ability, and all he could do was pass on his *own* cumulative understanding.

In the early 1980s, I talked to Rollin about an article I wanted to write presenting his ideas about health and healing to a lay audience. He was quite fine with me writing it, but he specifically instructed me not to use his, Sutherland's, or Still's name in the piece. This was not because there was any secret about where these ideas came from. But Dr. Becker was emphatic that the information was now mine to use.

At the time I was truly just a beginner, and it seemed a ridiculous stretch of the imagination for me to think of myself as having anything of my own to say. But he was clear; in his view the ideas and information did not belong to anyone; they did not belong to Becker or Sutherland or Still. So, of course, when I wrote the article I did as he had asked.

In the decades that followed, when I was called upon to teach Rollin Becker's work – I always held lightly the idea that I was teaching "Rollin Becker." That's what people wanted – and I was grateful for the opportunity to help preserve and pass along his valuable ideas and approaches. For years, I titled the course I taught as "The Legacy of Rollin Becker, DO" – I used the word "legacy" to emphasize that what I was teaching was my understanding and experience of what I had received. I always kept in mind the reality, and tried to make plain to others, that all I could be teaching was "Rachel Brooks." Around the time I turned 60, I finally dropped his name from my course titles acknowledging this reality, and I could picture Rollin nodding his head in approval with an amused smile on his face.

Professional Evolution

Jacques Duval, as told by Mark Baker

The first summer that Jacques was in Dallas, Rollin emphasized to him the importance of raising the energy level of the patient with your treatment. If the patient came in at a six, they should be at a seven when they went out. If they came in at a six and it went down to a five, then there was something not right in what you had done.

In the year that followed, back in Paris, Jacques worked very diligently to get so that he could accomplish this boosting of the energy with his treatments. When he returned to Dallas the next summer, he reported to Rollin that he felt good about the progress he had made – he was getting good at being able to raise the energy level of the patient. Rollin responded: "That doesn't interest me anymore. Actually, I'm interested in where the energy comes from."

I heard Jacques tell this story in multiple situations, both in his teaching and in our conversations over a meal. This experience had a really big impact on him and he took away a number of lessons from it.

On a practical level, Jacques emphasized that it is one of the goals in treatment to have lifted the energy of the patient, but more importantly we do not want to lower their energy through overtreatment. Jacques would tell us: "Do not treat patients to death." A story that goes along with this is: Rollin once asked Jacques to treat his knee, which Jacques did to the best of his ability. When Jacques was through, he said, "There you are Rollin." Rollin replied, "But the treatment was already finished ten minutes ago Jacques."

Then there was the meaning Jacques took from Rollin saying, "that no longer interests me." I see that as an exercise of being in the present. I believe Jacques taught the way Rollin taught him. He did not want to waste any time. He assumed that you got what he was talking about and that we can move on. Jacques also took those words as Rollin's way of saying "do not get stuck in your understanding; if you really can raise the patients' energy level, I am not going to pat you on the back. I expect you to go deeper."

This then leads to the aspect of professional evolution. Jacques was really enthused by this notion. He felt like his mission was to stay firmly in the principles described by Rollin, but also to push that knowledge as far as possible and to never stop. And out of love and respect towards Rollin, that is what Jacques did right up until he died in 2005. He said that as a student you have to fasten your seat belt and hang on to the coat tails. Learning, like teaching, is a dynamic changing adapting process. The student does not know how it will evolve, but to really learn he must be completely present in this evolution.

What Did He Mean?

Rachel Brooks

Whenever the topic of Dr. Becker's teachings comes up, there is one question I am invariably asked. That question is: What did Dr. Becker mean when he said [*fill in the blank*]? In response, there are times I feel confident I can answer the question with clarity. But often my answer is prefaced by saying something like: I don't *know* for sure, although I *believe* this is what he meant based on things I heard him say, saw him do, or experienced as he was working on me or others. Sometimes, I can only say, "I really don't know."

Whatever my response, I usually follow that by saying, "What I can tell you now is that this is my current understanding of what he meant based on my own knowledge and experience." It has always been important to me in my teaching to keep a clear distinction between what I *know* about what Dr. Becker thought and did and what my *interpretations* and further understandings have been.

It is now about 30 years since I was last able to communicate with Rollin, and I often think of all I would give to have the chance for one more conversation with him so that I could ask all these questions. In the years that I spent time with him, I was so relatively young, in age and in practice, that I did not even know the questions to ask, and I was not much of an asker of questions back then anyway. I just took in all that he offered to me – grateful to have been taken under his wing and given the opportunity to try and "stand on his shoulders" as he used to say.

There is so much I wish I knew from all the great osteopaths who came before me, but I know Dr. Becker would have been the first to respond to this notion by pointing out the reality that each of us is on our own journey of discovery. We can be bolstered and nourished by our teachers, but ultimately, we are challenged and free to make the work our own.

Some years ago, I was reading through old Sutherland Cranial Teaching Foundation documents and found the answer to one of the lingering questions I would have loved to ask him. The question I had was about Dr. Sutherland and his development of the cranial concept. In his 1964 President's Report, Dr. Becker wrote about the project of publishing Sutherland's collected works in what would eventually become the book *Contributions of Thought*.

> It is my opinion that the easiest way to assemble them would be for Adah [Sutherland] and Anne Wales to arrange them according to the timetable in which they appeared…. In this manner, it would point towards Dr. Will's continuous growth and development in his understanding as well as making it easier to put together. One important weakness of this approach is that Dr. Will knew about and used the Potency of the Cerebrospinal Fluid as he developed his understanding of the cranial concept in the period between 1900 and 1925 but he did not give us this information until 1946 or 1947. However, explanatory notes in the assembled material could clear this and other points as they arose.

I appreciated reading these words of Dr. Becker. I had known that Sutherland was using the Potency and Tide long before he felt it was the right time to teach it, but I didn't know how long that arc of time really had been. I had assumed that Sutherland's understanding of these things must have deepened over time, but it kind of reassured me that even for those we know of as great thinkers and explorers, it still took time for their wisdom and knowledge to grow. I often confess that it took me decades for my own understanding of Stillness to truly mature after Dr. Becker first instilled the importance of it in me.

What Still and Sutherland Knew

Jacques Duval, as told by Mark Baker

In the course of their conversations, Rollin told Jacques that Will Sutherland was sure that Dr. Still knew about these things; the things they were now exploring about the cranial mechanism. He said that Will was absolutely sure Still knew about them, but that Dr. Still understood it in an intuitive way and didn't have the time to fully understand it and find a way to articulate and teach it.

Jacques then asked if Sutherland knew all these things that Rollin was teaching him, and Rollin said the same thing. He said that Will knew it all, but that he did not have the time to completely understand and articulate it. For instance, Will had told Rollin that he did not *fully* understand the Breath of Life until the last year of his life.

Rollin concluded these remarks by saying: I have had so many more years to understand these things intellectually, to experience and articulate them, but I have not done a thing that Sutherland did not already know.

Without Judgment or Expectation

Thomas McCombs

It was 1988 when some of the greatest osteopathic masters alive assembled in Tulsa, Oklahoma for the Sutherland Cranial Teaching Foundation (SCTF) course. At the time, I was in my internship year. While at the course I experienced the joy, fellowship, and cultivation of skills found at other osteopathic gatherings – but here it was done with an unrivaled master-student focus.

Dr. John Harakal, the president of the SCTF at the time, shared in his lecture a description of his own brush with death and his response to osteopathy. Dr. Harakal told us how he had survived a massive myocardial infarction. In fact, his cardiac enzyme levels were higher than any other survivor of such an event who had been seen at Fort Worth Osteopathic Hospital. Found slumped over his desk at the Texas College of Osteopathic Medicine, Dr. Harakal had been taken across the street to the hospital and was slipping into cardiogenic shock when Dr. Rollin Becker arrived from Dallas. Dr. Becker declined to stop and review the EKG and labs and just threaded his way through the IV lines and EKG leads to Dr. Harakal's bedside.

Dr. Becker's description of what he did when he got to the bedside was: "I put my hands on the patient and listened without judgment or expectation." This statement was all he said about the osteopathy that he employed. We can never know for certain what role Dr. Becker's approach played, but after that treatment Dr. Harakal came out of cardiogenic shock. He not only survived, but he went on to recover and returned to academia until he succumbed to cerebrovascular disease a few years later.

After this presentation, Dr. Becker was aggressively questioned from the audience about "what specific techniques did you apply?" In response, he only repeated over and over again: "I put my hands on the patient and listened without judgment or expectation."

To see an osteopathic master boil down all the osteopathy they had ever delivered to that one principle went beyond me. Personally, I am an engineer of the living. I fix things. I do things to restore lost function. I craft and deliver specific osteopathic manipulative treatment, chosen from various models to match the patient's structural needs. I do not listen without judgment or expectation. Perhaps I should. Dr. Becker did.

Response of a Master

Michael Burruano

One of the first times I put my hands on a patient at a cranial course to discern motion and pattern, Rollin Becker was my table trainer. I looked up and said, "I feel it doing 'this,' but I don't know if it's him or me." He looked up at me with a slight smile and shrugged his shoulders. It took almost 30 years of practice and teaching for me to be able to respectfully answer a question in that manner – and to my surprise, it was not from knowing, but from the deepest sense of *not* knowing.

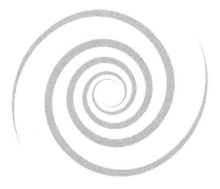

They Don't Get It

Caroline Tosh

Dr. Becker was very supportive of me, and I am grateful for all the bits of time I had with him. On his last visit to the UK in 1988, he presented his paper "Flexibility in Osteopathy" at a meeting, and it went very badly. By that time, he was really not functioning at 100 percent – I thought maybe he was getting hard of hearing. He refused to use a microphone and was a bit mumbly, so you had to really work to hear what he had to say. The audience was not very cooperative. In those days the cranial teaching was still really breaking ground in the UK. There were still people who wanted to be converted; people who didn't see that they needed to work to get to a place of understanding. These days you would have in the audience 200 people, all of whom would be hanging on every word.

Being there and watching this unfold, it was very sad and heartbreaking for me to watch. Dr. Becker was aware of this, and he seemed terribly sad as we walked back to the hotel together. He said to me: "They just don't get it; I don't know if they will ever get it."

As I think about it now, it is so wonderful that Anne Wales lived long enough to see her work carried on. That is not something Rollin ever got to see. He saw his work manifest in various individuals, but he did not see a wide understanding of what he was trying to teach. It must have been hard to work for so long and still wonder if it was ever going to go anywhere. By the time Dr. Becker expressed those feelings in 1988, I had become a table trainer, and I'd like to think that over the years as a faculty, we in the UK have contributed to anchoring his work here.

Editor's note: By 1988 Dr. Becker had begun to be affected by vascular dementia, and one of the greatest initial impacts from that condition for him was on his language capacities. That was the last year he did any formal teaching.

That Last Treatment

Rachel Brooks

In the late 1980s, Dr. Becker began having multiple small strokes, and because of this, he retired at the age of 79. After a while, he moved into a retirement community with his wife and in the early 1990s, I made a trip to visit with them. They had a small apartment there and in due course, Rollin requested that we get the portable treatment table set up.

At the time of that visit, Rollin was struggling with getting his words out in conversation and needed some help in getting things done. When we got the treatment table set up, he indicated he wanted to treat me. So, I got on the table, and it took him quite some time and effort to get himself settled properly into the chair. Then it took some more time and effort for him to get his hands arranged for the treatment. His hands ended up in some configuration that was not one of his usual holds, but eventually he was satisfied.

Then, Rollin began the treatment, and I

immediately felt his awareness shift and
I experienced what I had always felt as
the essence of his treatment. That is, this
extraordinary state of Stillness and the healing
potential manifested within. The room filled
with an experience of that profound state.
It was a powerful lesson for me in learning
about the nature of Stillness. Even with
his mind and motor skills compromised,
there was no diminution or alteration in
the state of Stillness. It was a poignantly
perfect example of how Stillness can never
be diminished; it is always there quietly and
beautifully expressing itself – an all-pervasive,
universal, state of energy.

That was the last treatment I would receive
from Dr. Becker, and I wouldn't trade that
experience for any treatment I have had since.
I felt such gratitude for all that he had given
to osteopathy and to me.

Robert C. Fulford, DO

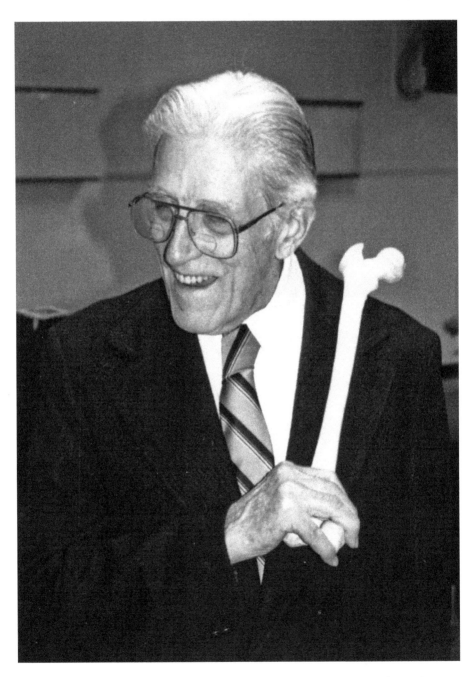

Robert Fulford pictured with a femur. This playful homage to the iconic picture of Dr. Still was taken by an osteopathic student who was also a professional photographer, at the Kirksville College of Osteopathic Medicine, circa 1990. Photo by Cary M. Bisbey, DO.

Robert C. Fulford, DO
(1905 – 1997)

Robert Fulford always wanted to be a physician. However, his fulfillment of that wish was delayed and shaped by unforeseeable obstacles. After completing college, he was to begin medical school in the fall of 1929, but with the stock market crash and Great Depression, this became impossible. Instead, Robert went to work in industrial plants to help support his family for six years. Eventually, after a significant work-related injury to his hand, he decided again to pursue a medical career. But that also did not go as planned. Though he had been promised a placement in the medical school, without a reason given, the dean said he thought he was better suited to being a dentist – and Robert walked away from this suggestion. Then a year later he learned about osteopathy from a friend and embarked upon the path that would be his life's calling. He graduated from the Kansas City College of Osteopathic Medicine in 1941.

While a student, Fulford's deep interest in studying the philosophical and spiritual principles of life and health was established. He absorbed A.T. Still's writings; became connected with the New Thought Movement; and began exploring the life sciences of the day that were beginning to demonstrate the nature of the "life energies." This exploration continued throughout his lifetime – he read widely and learned from many diverse types of healers and scientists.

In 1942, Fulford began his studies with Dr. Sutherland and continued studying with him throughout the 1940s. Dr. Fulford was deeply inspired by these studies, and they provided him with important knowledge and skills. He was also drawn to the work of Beryl Arbuckle, DO, including her research and innovative osteopathic work with children. He often traveled to Dr. Arbuckle's clinic in Pennsylvania to study with her.

While Sutherland and Arbuckle were major influences in the development of his treatment approach, Dr. Fulford continuously sought out other ideas and methods that could expand his understanding and help in restoring health to his patients. Robert, more than most of the other osteopathic practitioners of his day, openly embraced other disciplines and treatment approaches, and he more freely spoke of the spirit and energy inherent in Life and healing. In his searching over the years: he connected with people such as Dr. Randolph Stone, Dr. John Diamond, and Valerie Hunt, PhD; he keenly read the writings of Walter Russell and many others; and he incorporated into his practice ways of working that included the percussion vibrator (percussion hammer), magnets, and Vogel crystals.

His use of the percussion hammer is an example of Dr. Fulford's continual development. When he first took up its use, he applied it as a soft tissue treatment device to overcome the difficulty of treating highly stressed patients on the home front during World War II. Then, over time, he refined the percussion hammer's use from a soft tissue treatment device to one that can directly influence the life energy field.

Robert Fulford spent most of his practice life in Cincinnati, Ohio, then moved to Arizona in 1979. His intention was to retire there, but Robert was naturally inclined to help those who sought his help, especially children, and so he soon found himself busy with patients again. Finally, after about 10 years, seeking a true retirement from patient care he returned to Ohio.

Dr. Fulford was involved in teaching over many years. He was closely affiliated with the Osteopathic Cranial Academy where he served as president from 1974-75. He also taught courses with the Sutherland Cranial Teaching Foundation through the 1980s. Around that same time, he also began teaching his own courses. He taught courses on his approach to Energy Medicine and taught many on the use of the Percussion Hammer. In addition to his lectures and courses, over the years he welcomed many interested students and physicians into his practice and home.

Dr. Fulford was a gentle, humble, and quiet man. He encouraged all who studied with him to follow their passion and explore the wide uncharted paths in the study of Life, spirituality, and science; and to apply what they learned to their patients. This is what Dr. Fulford did throughout his lifetime until his death at the age of 91.

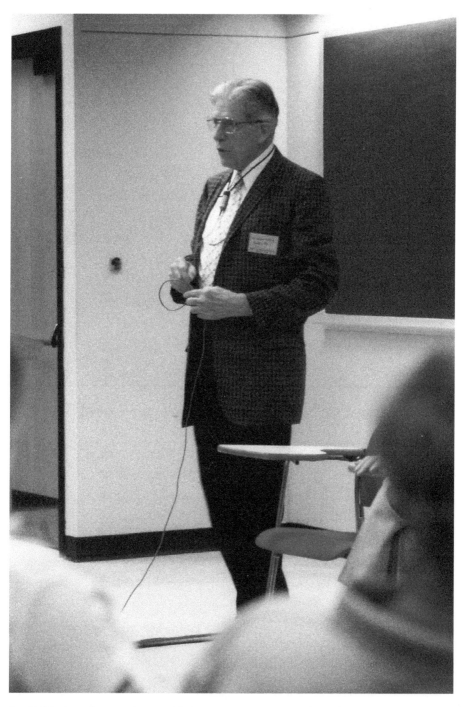

Dr. Fulford speaking at the 1984 SCTF course in Fort Worth at the Texas College of Osteopathic Medicine. Photo by Donald Becker, MD.

Let's Take Care of That

Paula Eschtruth

It was my great fortune to have had the relationship with Dr. Fulford that I did. At my first cranial conference in 1975, I was limping around with a really swollen knee and foot, having recently come out of a cast for a fractured talus. As I limped past this one instructor, he said, "Let's take care of that," and led me to a treatment table. He placed one hand on my ankle and one on my knee. It seemed like he did nothing but within hours the swelling was gone from my knee and ankle! That was my introduction to Dr. Fulford.

In that same conference, during one of the palpation sessions, the table trainer I had actually slapped my hands away, saying I was not feeling the right thing. Dr. Fulford saw this and afterwards he let me know that what I was feeling was really there. So began my relationship with Dr. Fulford – a relationship of mutual respect and kinship.

Love, Light, and Life

Richard Koss

Dr. Fulford lived and practiced Osteopathy only in the invisible world of Love, Light, and Life. Without having an awareness of the existence and reality of the energy fields it is difficult to comprehend the nature of Dr. Fulford's treatments. It seems to me that a great majority of physicians who encountered him attempted to fit Dr. Fulford's work into their own personal background, training, and the accepted modern scientific methods of research and practice. Doing this usually leads to false assumptions and conclusions as they attempt to explain how Dr. Fulford was able to produce such miraculous results. Often, when his students were unable to explain his methods or duplicate his results, he was called a "gifted healer" with "God-given gifts."

Dr. Fulford did not accept these descriptions. He thought this knowledge and its application was something all who worked at could attain. However, in order to accomplish this, they must be willing to leave their comfort zone of knowledge and challenge their tried-and-true methods and techniques. This is a major hurdle that limits so many. But, with determination, it is a hurdle that can be crossed over. And indeed, Dr. Fulford has had tremendous influence on several of the great osteopaths in our profession today. All of them that I know state that studying and spending time with Dr. Fulford literally changed their lives both personally and in their practices. They all reflect on how Dr. Fulford inspired them to study the timeless truths of Osteopathy as demonstrated by the example of his life. This quiet, humble, and great Osteopath certainly inspired me.

What Our Hands Tell Us

Paula Eschtruth

At some point, I began assisting Dr. Fulford in his courses, and somewhere in the midst of each course he would turn to me and say, "Paula, you show them this approach." I would then start to demonstrate and explain the approach just as I had seen him do it. But then he would always interrupt me and say, "No, not like that," and he would go on to show some different version of the technique.

It was unsettling at first. I knew I was teaching the approach just as I had seen him teach it. But what those experiences taught me was that Dr. Fulford was always responding to what the patient needed. And because what each patient needs is always different, our approach will always be different too. In this way Dr. Fulford taught me that our treatment is based on what our "thinking, feeling, knowing hands" tell us.

There It Is

Thomas Thrall

During a table session in Dr. Fulford's course on
his energy approaches, the instruction given was to
place our hand on the patient's abdomen in order
to perceive a particular thing that had just been
described. After a time, it became clear that no one in
the room was really getting it, and Dr. Fulford must
have picked up on the confused looks on all our faces.
At that time, he simply walked around the room,
going to each table in turn, and placed his hand over
each of ours, saying "There it is."

My experience, when he placed his hand over mine,
was like a television set had just been turned on;
everything that he had been talking about suddenly
came into focus and became quite clear. This taught
me a powerful lesson about levels of perception, that
a deeper and more profound treatment is always
possible if the physician is capable of perceiving the
mechanism on the level that it is actively working.

Tell Them Something

Rachel Brooks

Edgar Miller, DO, was a wonderful mentor and friend of mine in Boston who had graduated osteopathic school in 1953. Ed knew many of the greats of his own generation as well as those who were his elders, and he would often tell me stories about his experiences with them. Once, he told me a story, probably in the late 1980s, about an experience he had with Dr. Fulford. They were standing together at a conference and Dr. Fulford was approached by an attendee who asked him a question and a simple answer was given. Soon after this, another person approached and asked essentially the same question. Dr. Fulford responded with a decidedly different, but still simple, answer.

After this, Ed asked him how he could give such different and sort of contradictory answers to the same question. Dr. Fulford, with a wry smile and slight shrug of his shoulders, said something to the effect that: You have to tell them something; they want an answer; and in most cases it doesn't really matter what you say.

At the time, I was only a few years into teaching this work and was still absorbing so much from these mentors of mine about teaching. These words of Dr. Fulford's really struck me. From the way Ed told the story and from the time I had spent around Dr. Fulford at courses, I did not suspect that his intention was to lead anyone astray, dismiss them, or say anything that had no meaning. Instead, I think he was acknowledging that his words might keep a student thinking and engaged, and that ultimately each person needs to find their own way to their own understanding.

Always Something to Learn

Paula Eschtruth

Over the years, Dr. Fulford and I attended many different courses together. We would each keep our eye out for classes beyond osteopathy that sounded interesting, and when we found one, we then made plans to go together. The topics of these courses ranged widely including many different approaches to healing. The courses we took included:

Dr. Douglas Baker on esoteric healing; Marcel Vogel on love and crystal healing; Dr. John Diamond on energy healing and magnets; various offerings at the University of the Trees with Christopher Hills, Victoria Beasley, and Robert Massey; and the Healing Conference in Boulder, Colorado where many alternative healing methods were presented.

Dr. Fulford and I found there was always something to be learned in these classes that could help us in our practices.

My Silent Need to Know

Patrick Wedlake

One of the conditions that challenged me for a while in my practice was that after some traumas, I found the head of the femur was not quite settled into the acetabulum and I struggled to get this to resolve. The associated history was typically that the patient had slipped while all their weight was on one leg or some similar type of strain.

So, I diligently read and tried to duplicate the three variants of Dr. Still's techniques listed in his book, *Research & Practice*. None of them ever worked for me. Then I attended the Founder's Day Conference in Kirksville one year that honored Kim Korr, PhD (who had been my small group facilitator for two years at the Texas College of Osteopathic Medicine). Dr. Fulford was one of the speakers, and it was during a practical on the use of the percussion hammer that he looked straight at me and said, "And if you ever can't get a hip back in place, here's where you put the percussor...." And then he proceeded to demonstrate the procedure, which has been successful in my hands ever since.

At the time, I came away wondering, how is it that I am so transparent? I felt that it reflected some limitation or inadequacy in me. Now, I reflect that I was indeed transparent in my wish and Dr. Fulford remarkably responded to my silent need to know.

My Perception Was Altered

R. Paul Lee

When I had been practicing osteopathy in the cranial field for about five years, I had an important experience visiting Dr. Fulford in his Tucson office. I was standing across the treatment table while he was treating an infant using the percussion hammer. One hand was holding the hammer while the other was monitoring the effect in the baby's tissue. Unable to control my impulse, I reached out to touch his hands so that I might feel what he was observing. He looked up at me and said to me, "Don't do that; you'll short me out." Then, he offered, "Come around behind me and place your right hand on my right hand and your left hand on my left hand." When I did, in a moment, his treatment culminated in a release which was accompanied by him jumping.

My perception was altered after that experience. I was able to perceive more subtly. And I also began jumping, myself, rather randomly at first and with time reliably with the phases of treatment: engagement, unwinding, integration, still point, and return of easy normal motion. It was as if Dr. Fulford had inducted me into my true osteopathic being.

I was also impacted by Dr. Fulford's statement that we treat more effectively when we keep our minds focused on the task, rather than thinking about what we are going to do for dinner or afterward. He encouraged us to observe what is transpiring in the tissues and treat with the sense of love.

Get The Old Wheels Turning

Thomas Thrall

When I was a third-year medical student in Indianapolis (1975), I was first introduced to osteopathy by Dr. Rollin Becker. During that informal meeting, he gave me a brief treatment and suggested that I might want to connect and follow-up with Dr. Fulford in Cincinnati.

So, I made an appointment with Dr. Fulford, and in my initial treatment, as I lay on the table, he moved about my body checking out different things. During that process I do not recall feeling anything in particular. Then, he got his hands under my head, and I expected to feel something like the deeply quiet state that I had experienced when Dr. Becker had held my head for several minutes.

Instead, within a second, I experienced a great, electric blue ball shoot from the center my head, down through my body, and out the bottom of my feet. It seemed about the size of a melon. Dr. Fulford then calmly said, "There, that should get the old wheels turning."

Needless to say, this made a very big impression on me. It confirmed for me what I had already suspected from my initial contact with Dr. Becker, that this work was of a higher order, capable of creating deep change. The work had physical and mechanical aspects, but it also embodied things far beyond that. It seemed an exciting challenge to pursue this path of osteopathy.

My Spiritual Side

Michael Burruano

While I was in my first year of osteopathic practice and using HVLA (high velocity-low amplitude) for all my osteopathic treatments, I attended the American Academy of Osteopathy convocation where I was first introduced to Robert Fulford, DO. I recognized that he was esoteric, knowledgeable, and of some professional stature, but I was, for some reason, not shy about approaching someone who I thought could answer my questions.

During that conference, I approached him at a time when he was sitting by himself and asked if I could ask him a couple of questions. He complied and I said, "I tell my patients that it is OK to suffer. I know it is, but I'm not sure of the explanation why?" He said, "Oh, you didn't listen to my lecture; suffering tempers the soul to accept higher spiritual understanding." Though I indeed had not heard that in his lecture [Ugh!], I recognized those words from somewhere in my own experience. I then asked, "Then why bother healing – trying to help people get well?" He replied something to the effect that it is to allow people to be around long enough to know and have relationship with God. I appreciated being able to ask these kinds of questions which I had been pondering.

Later, when he was awarded an honor, I think at this same conference, Dr. Fulford responded, "I want to thank osteopathy for teaching me how to love." That statement impressed me. It was further confirmation that there was a lot more to this practice of osteopathy than just what our hands were doing.

And so, osteopathy stimulated my spiritual side, even in my HVLA practice. My first osteopathic sense of "Stillness" was observed positioning patients for a lumbar HVLA as my teachers, Drs. Nicholas S. Nicholas and David Heilig, had taught. I was reminded of that Stillness years later when Anne Wales asked me if I had ever noticed how sometimes, during a treatment, the whole room goes still? I give thanks for my teachers who taught from different perspectives, that "treatment" was always in the (Still) moment, within the need of the patient, gentle, and specific.

Bring the Soul in Contact

Thomas Thrall

There is one thing that Dr. Fulford said that moved me more than anything else. He was speaking at a conference in 1985 on the treatment of children and was emphasizing the importance of the breath. Then, in his concluding remarks, he stated, "The art of the healer is to bring the soul in contact with the body, and to give, in a loving way, unto that body, its purpose and reason to live. Then, the body can heal itself."

This spoke to me deeply in that moment and became a guiding principle for my treatments and for my own spiritual work over the years.

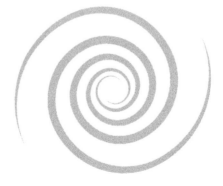

Be on a Higher Level

Thomas Thrall

In the 1980s, I took one of Dr. Fulford's "Energy" courses. In it, he explained his understanding that a patient comes to you with a problem which may exist on a particular level: physical, mental, emotional, etheric, or cosmic. He told us that one needs to be able to recognize the level on which the patient's problem resides, to be able to resolve it most effectively. Some problems are purely mechanical, and can be resolved with a simple adjustment, but often the imbalance goes deeper and must be addressed there. He added that the physician always needs to be present in their awareness on a level above the problem, in order to be able to perceive fully what is going on.

As part of the discussion of how we, as physicians, could prepare ourselves to do this work, Dr. Fulford explained his personal program. He shared his own understanding of *tithing*, stating that we were not being asked to tithe money, but it was 10% of our time that we were called upon to give. He then set aside two and a half hours daily for meditation and exercise to clear and vitalize his body and energy so he could be of service.

I had a meditation practice going at the time, but his words certainly brought new depth and meaning to it, showing me that it could be of immense practical value in my treatment of patients.

Frozen Shoulders and Intention

Thomas Thrall

I twice experienced Dr. Fulford's remarkable capacity to resolve frozen shoulders. In one of the demonstrations he gave, I knew the person with the frozen shoulder personally. At the time, the man could not lift his arm more than 20 degrees.

As an observer, what I saw was that with the patient standing, Dr. Fulford placed one hand on his arm and one on top of the shoulder. Then he had the patient take a breath deep into their abdomen, hold it for a bit to concentrate their resolve, and then breathe out forcefully through their nose. Dr. Fulford then simply lifted the patient's arm comfortably overhead.

Following this demonstration, Dr. Fulford spoke of the importance of intention, and of how a focused, forceful breath out through the nose can be used as a way to release and clear resistance in a treatment. Certainly, he was able to demonstrate that remarkably well!

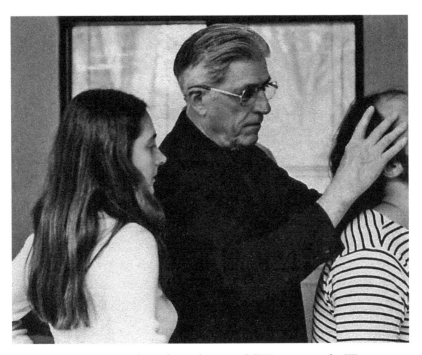

Dr. Fulford with Jayne Alexander at the 1980 SCTF course at the West
Virginia College of Osteopathic Medicine. Photo by Mark Rosen, DO.

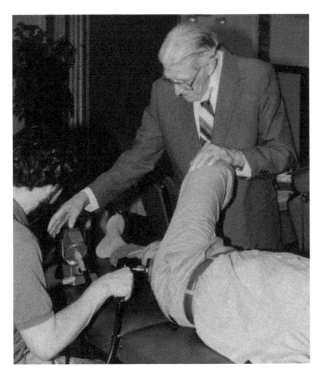

Dr. Fulford teaching
a Percussion Hammer
course in Tucson,
instructing Eric Dolgin,
in the early 1990s.

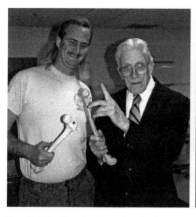 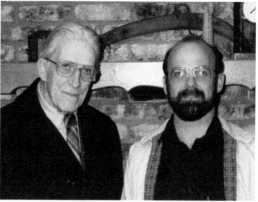

Dr. Fulford with Cary M. Bisbey
at the Kirksville College of
Osteopathic Medicine, circa 1990.

Dr. Fulford with Richard Koss, 1994.

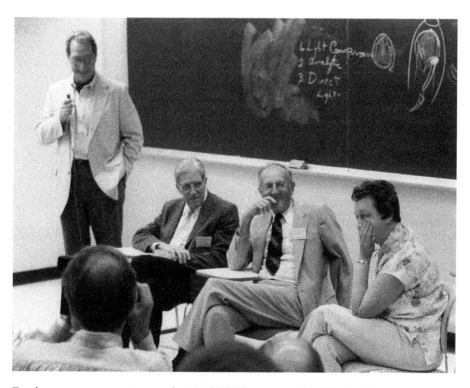

Faculty answering questions at the 1984 SCTF course in Fort Worth, Texas.
Left to Right: Herbert Miller, Robert Fulford, Rollin Becker, Edna Lay.
Photo by Donald Becker, MD.

Go Where the Problem Is

Thomas Thrall

Here are two stories I heard from Dr. Edgar Miller: At one of our occasional study group meetings in the Boston area, probably in the late 1980s or early 90s, Ed shared a couple of his stories about Robert Fulford. Once, while at a conference, Ed had a very bad headache and was just standing around when he saw Dr. Fulford approaching. Dr. Fulford walked up to him, stepped on his foot, and said something like: "I thought you might want someone to take care of that cuboid." And Ed's headache went away.

Another time, after a cranial course, Dr. Fulford was treating one of the participants. Dr. Fulford began by placing his hands down by the feet for a few minutes, then he came around to the side of the table, had the patient get on their side, and to Ed's surprise, he did an HVLA (high velocity low amplitude) lumbar roll.

These stories made an impression on me. The cuboid story was a good reminder that where the symptoms are and where the cause resides might be a far distance apart. The other story, of Dr. Fulford using an HVLA approach in a cranial course setting, was a good reminder that it matters less what technique you use as long as you get the job done well. Both stories seemed to be guidance to go to where you perceive the problem is and do what you are inclined to do to remedy it.

It's All Connected

Bonnie Gintis

When I was still an osteopathic student,
I attended an "Evening With The Stars"
at the American Academy of Osteopathy
convocation. Various participants or members
of their families presented themselves to Dr.
Fulford for his evaluation and treatment. His
handling of these "patient" encounters taught
me some lasting lessons.

There was a woman with depression seeking
help. After evaluating her and asking her
about the crystal necklace she was wearing,
Dr. Fulford concluded the crystal was the
problem. He told her that she would be fine
if she stopped wearing the necklace or had the
crystal re-set into an orientation that would
be in harmony with her energy field. He did
not treat her at all, and he explained why: "If
I treat you, you will think it was the treatment
that helped."

Dr. Fulford next saw a toddler with frequent
ear infections. He did a brief exam and then
asked to see him walk. When the child was
back on the table, he showed us the tibial
torsion in one leg, explained that the fibula was
the actual problem, and proceeded to sort it

out in short order. He told the father, "I think that's all he's going to need for his ears to clear up" (which I know is true because I asked the father about it a year or two later). Dr. Fulford then told us that he didn't want us to think his identification of the fibula as the problem was magic or somehow mystical, and so he went on to trace the anatomy from the fibula, up through the pelvis and all the way to the cranial base. The temporal bone was indeed affected, he said, but if you only treated the cranium the fibula would keep re-creating the lesion.

This experience was really important for me as a student, particularly since I was in a newcomer's honeymoon phase with the cranial concept – sitting at the head of the table believing it was the way to solve all problems. Dr. Fulford showed how everything really is connected – connected both within the body as well as to things outside the body. It was a great lesson in not letting yourself get stuck in a box, like the cranial box, and the importance of finding the true cause of the problem. It helped me not to expect to find the solution in any one place; and not to forget the rest of the body and everything else that influences health.

A Release From Trauma

Caroline Tosh

I have to admit I didn't really understand Dr. Fulford's teachings when I first heard them at a Sutherland Cranial Teaching Foundation course in the UK in the early 1980s. As a student on that course, I wasn't sure what to make of his talk of mind, body, and spirit being triune and things like that. But at the end of the course, I had a rather important treatment from him. It is quite a story how that came to pass.

It had become commonplace for me that by the end of a cranial course, I was physically and emotionally a wreck. This sensitivity was not surprising as I had a history of a bad injury in a swimming pool that resulted in a brain trauma and C1 fracture when I was 16 years old. After this course, when my husband came to pick me up, I rushed into his arms and burst into tears. He said, "Oh no, not again," and asked where the faculty were having their post-course meeting. He went over to where I pointed, knocked on the door and told the course director, "I'm tired of picking her up and her being in a heap. She was in perfectly good shape when I brought her down here and I want her back the same way!" In response, Colin Dove, the course director asked Dr. Fulford if he would be willing to treat me.

So, this is how I got the treatment from Dr. Fulford. The treatment he gave me was not the gentle approach

I was used to. It hurt; it hurt a lot. He worked on pressure points in the pelvis and around the rib cage. He held me in place with these points and I felt like I couldn't breathe at all until I took a big gasp. I could then breathe and felt better, and when he finished, I could really breathe. And so my husband took me home. Then, three weeks later, I had a powerful, cathartic dream related to the head injury. And after that I felt very different with a sense of being "like my old self" from before the injury.

This experience alerted me to the knowledge that osteopathy can change more than just the physical. My treatment from Dr. Fulford brought not only a physical change, it brought a release from the trauma that was being carried in my being since the accident.

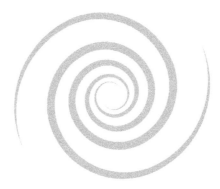

A Visceral Experience

Bonnie Gintis

Mid-way through my first Sutherland Cranial Teaching Foundation cranial course I developed pneumonia. In 1983, I had arrived in Colorado Springs for the course with a cold, which got steadily worse. By the third day it was clear I had pneumonia. That night in the hotel, my roommate, Mary Elizabeth Hitchcock, a 72-year-old DO from New York City, stayed up all night with me, treating me with various osteopathic approaches. Despite this dedicated care, come the morning I was beginning to turn blue and it was becoming more difficult to talk due to my shortness of breath, and so she alerted the faculty that we were heading for the hospital.

Dr. Fulford heard this and said something like, "Nobody in a course of mine goes to the hospital until I've treated them." So, while somebody was lecturing up at the front of the room, I was on a treatment table in the back. Over the next two and a half hours I had treatment from Bob Fulford, Rollin Becker, Gerry Slattery, and Edgar Miller. At times, it was one or the other of them, at others it was two, three, or all four of them. They all agreed it was a pneumonia in the right middle lobe.

Eventually, there was a moment when I actually felt my fever break. I felt something shift, like a veil was pulled away from my eyes, which came along with the thought "Oh, I'm back." They all felt it too. It was clear something had shifted. Suddenly I could breathe and my face turned pink. I spent the rest of that day propped up with a bunch of pillows, half-reclining, and listening to the lectures from a treatment table against the wall at the back of the room. Every hour or so one of them would come by and offer some kind of treatment. By the next day, I was well enough to participate in the course. I had some residual symptoms for a few weeks after that – but recovered steadily and well.

I was just a second-year osteopathic student at the time, and this was a powerful demonstration for me of what was possible using osteopathic treatment and what it feels like to receive treatment. In the osteopathic educational setting, students are largely working on each other's relatively healthy bodies and the kind of experience I had just doesn't happen in the school labs or even in the hospitals. This episode also led me, in my teaching, to always tell students in labs that I believe the person who does the most learning is the person lying on the table. That is because the person on the table gets to be quiet and feel what's happening, and they don't need to be worried about "Am I doing this right?" or "Am I feeling the right thing?"

I have always been very grateful for the extraordinary personal lesson in anatomy, physiology, pathology, and osteopathy all rolled into one that was offered up by these incredibly experienced people. On that day, I got to have a "visceral" experience of what it means to be treated osteopathically.

About That Scar

Chris Laseter

I was taking a course from Dr. Fulford as a young practitioner in the early 1990s, and in that course, he asked if he could demonstrate on me. While walking towards the table, Dr. Fulford said to the class, "You see there's the scar, and we're going to release the contents of the abdomen out of the pelvis." He had me position myself on the table, in the knee-chest position, with my rear end up in the air. He placed his percussion hammer on my coccyx, reached a hand up to the suprapubic area, and provided some cephalic traction. As he finished, I was aware of some release.

He explained that his treatment had disimpacted the ptotic abdominal contents from the true pelvis as a way of relieving my once-compromised appendiceal artery. He added that while this treatment was addressing an old, chronic condition in me, osteopaths had managed subacute appendicitis this way in earlier times. The implication being that this ptosed situation (where part of the intestine has sagged into the true pelvis) is a potential cause of appendicitis.

When I stood up, I noticed that this ptosis had lifted. Something had shifted; something that had existed since having a ruptured appendix many years before. However, I did not make much of it at that time. The importance of the lesson was lost upon me at that stage in my training. I later learned to manage subacute appendicitis in select patients using this principle. My management includes relieving ptosis of the cecum and lifting the pelvic floor using Sutherland's approach.

Only some years later did I realize that Dr. Fulford never lifted my shirt to observe the scar. He had never seen or palpated the scar that he told the class about, nor did he know of my history of appendicitis. I was astonished by his powers of perception. His sensitivity and awareness continue to inspire me today.

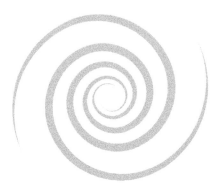

The Incredible Changes

Richard Koss

I, like many others, often share the case histories of treatments we observed Dr. Fulford giving. It is hard for those who listen to these case histories, as well as for those who observed them, to fully appreciate the meaning and depth of understanding the cases revealed.

In Doc's book, *Dr. Fulford's Touch of Life*, the ghost writer, Gene Stone, accurately described the case studies as they were told to him by Dr. Fulford. However, having personally witnessed or assisted in the vast majority of those treatment sessions, I feel the descriptions do not convey the incredible changes that took place. This is not surprising, as Dr. Fulford reported these case histories for the book in his usual humble way. He felt that these were typical osteopathic treatments and were no "big deal"; that they were the natural result of understanding and using the healing forces available to us all.

In the almost ten years I spent traveling with him and assisting him in his work, I witnessed so many incredible and seemingly miraculous treatments, I wish I could share all of them with the profession. Robert C. Fulford, DO was truly a great healer – I believe he was an Osteopath of Dr. A.T. Still's philosophical teachings and view of life. Like Dr. Still, Dr. Fulford was an explorer for Truth, willing to think outside the limits of modern medicine. He proved his life's work by the results achieved in the treatment room. The case studies, witnessed and described here, are proof of this great Osteopath's life and how he continues to inspire all who will venture into Dr. Fulford's world.

Becoming a Child

Richard Koss

The following is my first experience with Dr. Fulford treating one of my patients. "Frank" was an 18-month-old boy who had a foot turned inward. I was just finishing my residency in Osteopathic Manipulative Medicine in Kirksville and had taken Fulford's Percussion Hammer course twice. The patient's family were friends of my family and they lived in Kirksville. Even though the Kirksville College of Osteopathic Medicine (KCOM) had been there for generations, there remained skepticism between the townspeople and the "Osteopaths on the other side of the railroad tracks" and they were not always eager to seek osteopathic care.

Frank was all boy and very active! His left foot was so turned in that his pediatrician had referred him to Shriners Hospital in St. Louis, a four-hour drive away. Upon his return, Frank had a plaster cast on his lower leg, and he was to return weekly for several months for the foot to be turned straight. Not surprisingly, Frank was a mess. He was crying and was unable to walk, run, or play. His father, who was a carpenter and generally a fix-anything kind of guy, was devastated by the sight of his son crying as he dragged his casted foot around. So, he cut the cast off and finally agreed to have Frank see the "Osteopaths" at KCOM.

Frank's first visit in my office was a disaster. Accompanied by his mom and older sister, Frank would not sit still; he just kept running around the treatment room. Any attempt to corral him and put him on the table did not work as he wiggled out of any handhold and ran off – he would not let me evaluate or treat him. This happened a second time two weeks later. We then set up a third and final attempt to try and treat him before they were to take him back to St. Louis for the serial casting.

The morning of this third visit, I ran into Dr. Fulford, who was visiting with Dr. Gerry Slattery. I was desperate to get Frank treated and so I got up the courage to ask Dr. Fulford if he would help me treat little Frank. I briefly explained his condition and he agreed. So that afternoon after mom, sister and Frank were put in the treatment room, Dr. Fulford and I entered. Frank was doing his usual activity of being quite busy and constantly moving while Dr. Fulford went over to introduce himself to mom.

Dr. Fulford then bent down and started having a conversation with Frank's older sister. This went on for at least five minutes. I was confused, thinking that Dr. Fulford was going to treat Frank's sister. I quietly went over to them and whispered in Dr. Fulford's ear that the patient was the boy. He slightly turned his head towards me and whispered, "I know!" with a stern whisper and look. He then went back to talking to the sister for another minute or so. It seemed like an eternity as Frank was busy buzzing around the treatment room. Dr. Fulford then turned his attention towards Frank and introduced himself. He then asked Frank if he could climb up on the treatment table, which he did immediately!

Frank then proceeded to remain quiet and calm for almost 20 minutes as Dr. Fulford evaluated him and treated him using the percussion hammer. Dr. Fulford worked on his left knee but spent much of the treatment on his left hip, pelvis, and ribcage. When the treatment was over, Frank ran out of the treatment room and sprinted down the long hallway to the waiting room with *both toes facing forwards.* His left foot was only slightly turned in – it was at least 90% corrected. Frank never went back to the Shriners Hospital and grew up to be a strong and healthy boy.

Dr. Fulford said that the problem was in his hip and pelvis and not the knee and tibia as was the thinking of the time. And he said you must play with the child, becoming one yourself, if you want to be able to treat them. The fact that Frank climbed up on the table and sat still was amazing. And that the condition was corrected with one visit is something that I will never forget. It changed my life!

First Breath at Any Age

Richard Koss

At a Basic Percussion Hammer Course in Ft. Worth, Texas, there was a patient demonstration with a seven-year-old girl who had steroid-dependent asthma. Her asthma was severe – she had a Cushingoid appearance from the huge doses needed, and she had missed so much school that she likely would have to repeat second grade. She had previously been quite active and loved to play soccer, but now she could not even go outside to play at all. She was in the Emergency Department at least once a week and was hospitalized about once a month.

This was the basic history that was given to Dr. Fulford. She was small for her age and not obese. She willingly climbed up on the treatment table, and we observed that her breathing was so shallow that you could hardly see her chest move. Dr. Fulford worked on her legs, sacrum and spine with the percussion hammer and worked on her cranium with his hands. Next, Dr. Fulford used the percussion hammer on her rib cage from the right mid-axillary line area to treat the diaphragm. After about a minute you could see her thorax tighten up and she could hardly breathe, then her knees and arms flexed slightly before she took an enormous breath and lay flat breathing deeply. We could see her chest and abdomen rise.

As I was this child's physician (she was a classmate of my son and her family were neighbors), Dr. Fulford asked me to check on her in about a month. I did that, and remarkably she was off all her asthma drugs, and she was playing outside and had signed up for soccer. She did not need any further treatments and did not miss another day of school that year. In fact, she graduated high school never having had another asthma attack.

Dr. Fulford explained to me that this little girl did not properly get her first breath at birth. The miracle I witnessed was a seven-year-old finally getting her first breath of life. We all witnessed her official first breath – essentially her birthday. It demonstrated to me the importance of the birth process and the power of the "first breath" in each patient no matter how old they are. I learned to pay very close attention to the breath because it reflects the health and well-being of the person. As the breath is freed up, it reflects the progress in healing and anchors the changes in all aspects of the person. The witnessing of this case made a profound impact on me personally and professionally. I am so grateful to have had this opportunity to witness Dr. Fulford treat in such a powerful and profound way, and yet remain a quiet and humble human being.

The "Flip" in the Energy Field

Richard Koss

In the many years I spent with Dr. Fulford, I often witnessed a sudden shake or twitch of his hands at the moment of release during a treatment. I observed this in most of his treatments – some of these movements were large in scope while others were just a subtle shift that was barely visible. (This phenomenon was captured on film in Dr. Andrew Weil's 1987 video on YouTube: "Robert C. Fulford, DO, An Osteopathic Alternative.") Dr. Fulford described this as a "flip in the energy field" occurring as the tissue normalizes, releasing the traumatic energy.

In reference to this, I often heard other practitioners comment that Dr. Fulford's twitch or shake at that moment was only for show and was not a real experiential phenomenon. I suspect that these comments were due to the fact that very few osteopaths have been able to duplicate this. My own experience back then, as someone fairly new to Dr. Fulford's world of the energy field, was that I felt the tissues – the energy in the fascia – "wind up" but I did not really experience the actual "flip in the tissues."

This all changed in a patient demonstration at the end of a Percussion Hammer course in Ft. Worth, Texas. The patient was a young boy, about 10 years of age, who had come with his mother from Oklahoma to be seen by Dr. Fulford. I am not sure of the original diagnosis, but I remember the young boy was quite agitated and wiggly and because of that Dr. Fulford had me gently steady the boy's feet while the mother sat by her son's side with a reassuring hand on his chest. The boy slowly settled down as the treatment proceeded.

When Dr. Fulford used the percussion hammer on the boy's shoulder to release his occiput, I felt the tissues of both lower legs and feet becoming more tense, strongly winding up. Then in a sudden burst, something came down his legs like a rushing bolus of water, and it hit my hands with such force that my hands all but came off his feet. It was so dramatic that the mother's hands were pushed off her son's chest at the same time. She let out a startled scream and turned to Dr. Fulford and said very loudly: "What have you done to my son?" Meanwhile, the boy was lying on the table very calmly and peacefully with a grin on his face and a look of bliss. When he got up his entire facial features had changed.

So, at that moment, I knew that Dr. Fulford was truly treating in the energy field around and within the human body, and that he could generate an enormous amount of energy to release the traumas of life. I experienced first-hand that this energy is real and very palpable and that at the moment of release there truly is a "flip in the tissues."

Work in the Energy Fields

Richard Koss

Dr. Fulford never stopped reading and studying. Late in life, he was able to meet Marcel Vogel, who was a great inventor for the IBM corporation. In his retirement Vogel was given the research equipment he had used while at IBM and was able to work out how to get a tremendous amount of energy out of a quartz crystal. Having worked out the cutting and polishing process to get the energy focused, Vogel then applied this knowledge in the use of quartz crystals in healing.

Dr. Fulford attended one of Vogel's crystal healing courses and later went to the laboratory where Vogel recorded the energy generated by Dr. Fulford using the percussion hammer on the patient. The significant energy changes were recorded in both the patient and Dr. Fulford at the moment of release during treatment. This reassured Dr. Fulford that his lifetime of study and practice in the energy field was real and legitimate – even though mainstream medicine, including most of the osteopathic profession, were still not on that path. It also showed that the other pioneers in the healing arts including Still, Sutherland, Arbuckle, Rollin Becker, and others, were on the right track.

In his last presentation at the 50th anniversary conference of the Cranial Academy, Dr. Fulford demonstrated a new treatment procedure he had just worked out. He then admonished the osteopathic profession and especially the Cranial Academy (who have stayed close to Dr. Still's philosophy), to get back to the work in the energy fields otherwise the "medics will take you over." This was incredibly difficult for Dr. Fulford to say, as he would ordinarily never say a negative or unkind word. He agonized over this lecture for several years. This is why he did not allow any taping or recording of this lecture. He passed away 6 days later in 1997 at the age of 91 ½.

I had so many extraordinary experiences in the years I spent traveling with Dr. Fulford and assisting him in presenting his work, and I wish I could share all of them with the profession. He told me many times that he could not wait for the 21st century as the information and revelations coming ahead would be amazing and incredible, proving the truth of the timeless principles of life and healing discovered by A.T. Still, and demonstrated by the students of Still's Osteopathy.

Love and Intention

Zina Pelkey

In the late 1990s, I spent a day with Dr. Fulford a few weeks before he gave what was to be his final presentation. He was working on his lecture for the Cranial Academy annual conference and told me it would be the last thing he was going to do. Doc told me he was going to "drop a bomb on the Academy and talk about energy medicine." In his presentation, he advised us to delve into energy work with the warning: "Osteopathy will be left in the dust if it does not delve into the understanding of energy."

At the end of his presentation, a participant was brought to the stage for treatment. She was visibly gray, weak, and rather limp. Dr. Fulford then used his Vogel crystal, performing something he called the "Ring of Fire." Not surprisingly, she pinked up and her revived vitality was obvious to the audience.

There were many questions from the audience, including one that asked, "How would you suggest I start using one of those crystals?" As if it was the crystal that did the treatment! Dr. Fulford, who was then in his 90's, had a dry sense of humor. His answer to that question was something like this: "Well, for the past 40 years or so I have been getting up early in the morning and spending several hours or more in meditation and exercise – that's a good way to start."

Most people are not as disciplined as Dr. Fulford. Folks are more caught up in getting things done quickly and easily rather than facilitating the profound shifts that his treatments could enable. He was always seeking deeper understandings and more effective ways to help his patients. He studied many world philosophies and approaches to health and personal development. The exercises he used came from the East and the West, and they included all sorts of ancient knowledge. This was how he reached the level of inner peace and connectedness necessary to engage the piezoelectric forces in the crystal to resonate with the inner forces in each patient to bring about optimal well-being.

Dr. Fulford emphasized treating patients with "pure intention and unconditional love." Vogel crystals were cut with love and the intention of healing. I believe that there are universal truths that underlie the organized connectedness of everything. When we work with respect for these powerful forces, balance and health pervade.

Paying Our Respects

Richard Koss

At Dr. Fulford's gravesite, a small group gathered to pay our last respects as he was lowered into the ground. This was in June 1997. I knew all the people gathered except for two white-haired ladies. We all took turns and spoke of our great gratitude and love for a most humble yet inspiring healer and teacher. When it was time for these two elderly women to speak, they introduced themselves and said they had been teachers in a school for special-needs children in Cincinnati.

They described how their class was full of highly active and unruly kids that could not be in the regular classroom. In today's terms they would be classified as ADD/ADHD. The best that they could describe a typical day in their classroom with 12 hyperactive children was as pandemonium, chaos, and carnage. Children were jumping off desks; nothing could be placed on the walls for it would be ripped down and ripped up; and there was constant fighting.

Dr. Fulford's love of children and his commitment to them was such that he volunteered, free of charge, to come into their classroom and treat several of the children. These women said that every time Dr. Fulford came into their classroom all the children would go to their desks and sit quietly still for some time. This happened *every* time he would arrive. Several of the children treated by Dr. Fulford calmed down enough to rejoin their classmates in the regular school.

Please remember that Dr. Fulford moved away from Cincinnati in 1978 and this was in 1997. These retired schoolteachers were so impressed with Dr. Fulford that they found their way to his gravesite to honor and pay their last respects. As I listened to the elderly teachers recount their experiences with Dr. Fulford, I was not surprised as I had witnessed many amazing, miraculous results in the ten years I spent learning and helping him teach his work in Osteopathy. It struck me that the influence Doc had over his many years of practice, on so many people who would not really remember him, like those children described by the teachers, was truly astounding. I listened and realized that his personal influence on patients and Osteopathy was over. To realize that this quiet, humble, loving physician would care for these forgotten kids and make such a difference in their lives was truly the mark of a great man.

These teachers experienced this greatness and came to give their grateful thanks. We all felt the genuine love that was so typical of any encounter with Dr. Fulford. The grief and sorrow were overwhelming as I realized that his quiet demeanor, love and patience in giving me lessons in life, Osteopathy, and spirituality were over now. Like these teachers, I too experienced the greatness of a most remarkable physician. And as I looked around there were no dry eyes in the group as we all felt his presence among us. I still think of him every day and miss him very much.

Anne L. Wales, DO

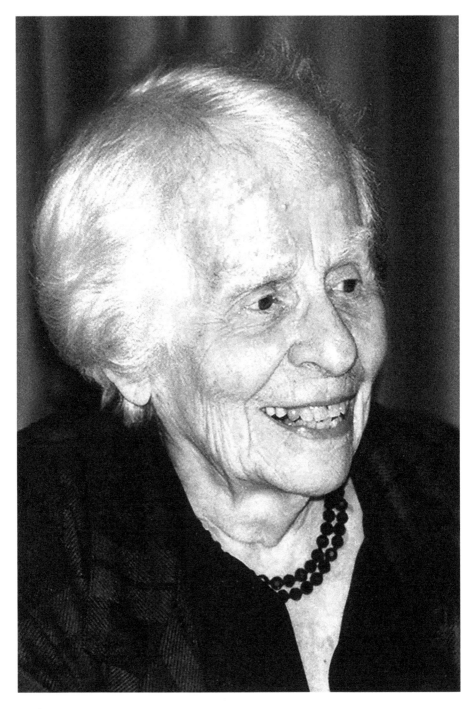

Anne Wales celebrating her birthday at a gathering organized by members of A Still Sutherland Study Group, mid-1990s. Photo by Michael Burruano, DO.

Anne L. Wales, DO
(1904 – 2005)

Anne Wales was born and raised in Rhode Island. Her connection to osteopathy began when she was a youth, after her mother was trampled by a horse and carriage. This accident left her mother in a painful disabled state, and whatever relief she was able to find came from the hands of a local osteopath. For Anne's osteopathic education: she traveled in 1922 from New England to Kirksville Missouri, later transferred to the Kansas City College of Osteopathic Medicine, and graduated from that school in 1926. After her internship, she returned to Rhode Island and practiced there until she retired in 1981 – at which time she moved to southern Massachusetts.

Dr. Wales had a deep and abiding connection with the natural world. Growing up by the large ocean bays of Rhode Island, she had an attunement to the rhythms and power of the forces of nature. She also had an attunement to greater forces – with a life-long interest in and connection with spiritual matters. Anne was an independent woman, willing to stand for herself and speak her mind when needed. In the early 1940s she married Chester Handy, DO, and together, in 1942, they first studied with Dr. Sutherland. From that time onward, their professional lives were focused on learning, teaching, promoting, and practicing Sutherland's work of osteopathy in the cranial field.

Amongst their many endeavors, Drs. Wales and Handy sponsored Dr. Sutherland in teaching courses in their home and became part of his teaching faculty. They dedicated much effort to the care of handicapped children: establishing a free clinic for treating these children and helping to organize schools. Over the years they served the Sutherland Cranial Teaching Foundation and Osteopathic Cranial Association in various ways: as founders, teachers, and board members. After Sutherland's death in 1954, Anne and Sutherland's wife, Adah, worked to collect his writings into a book that eventually became *Contributions of Thought*.

Following the sudden death of her husband in the early 1960s, Dr. Wales largely withdrew from traveling and teaching cranial courses. She said that Rollin Becker would occasionally coax her out to teach – but mainly she stayed home and tended to her osteopathic practice. In the early 1980s, after she had retired and moved to Massachusetts, a small trickle of young osteopathic students and practitioners found their way to her home and she would meet with them, teach them, and treat them. Over time, the numbers of those seeking her teaching grew, and in 1996 a group of them formed the "A Still-Sutherland Study Group" which has gone on to become a long-standing forum for her teaching.

In the 1980s, Dr. Wales also undertook the project of getting Dr. Sutherland's teachings – his spoken words – into a book. For seven years, Anne worked on this project that came to fruition with the publication of *Teachings in the Science of Osteopathy.* In this book and in all her teachings, she endeavored to be precise whenever she could. This was partly because it suited the workings of her mind, but also, she wanted those she taught to accurately understand what Sutherland had taught to her. While Sutherland's teachings were always at the core of her own teaching, Anne also freely shared her own experiences, insights, and new understandings.

Dr. Wales often expressed gratitude for the opportunities she had to pass these teachings on to younger generations. In the 1980s she shared with some of those who came knocking at her door, that she had been afraid she would die without passing on to others what Dr. Sutherland had given to her. Little did she know at the time that for the next twenty years she would teach and deeply impact a wide group of people from near and far. Anne continued to teach and inspire those around her until almost her last days when she died at the age of 101.

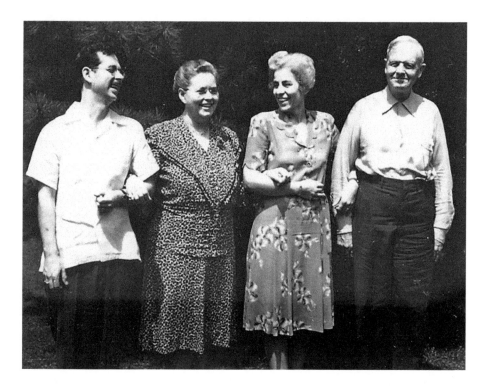

Left to Right: Chester Handy, Adah Sutherland, Anne Wales, and Will Sutherland in Moorestown, New Jersey, where Rebecca and Howard Lippincott lived. The Lippincott's were two prominent members of Dr. Sutherland's teaching faculty, and for years they led a study group that was an important source of support and learning to many. For five years, beginning in November 1944, Chester and Anne traveled from Rhode Island to attend the monthly study group, until the Lippincott's encouraged them to establish the New England Cranial Study Group.

Immovable Mountain

Sue Turner

I visited Anne's home during one of my visits to New England in the early 1990s. I had recently been in a highly stressful situation and my disturbance must have shown because after only five minutes of chatting, she announced, "I need to beat you up!"

Being accustomed to her sense of humor. I understood that this was her way of saying she was going to treat me. As she sat beside me, hands under my supine rib angles and fingers at the costovertebral junctions, (in the same way that she had treated pneumonia patients as an intern in the 1920s), she waited for the easing in the sympathetic chain ganglia. It felt as if she was connected to the center of the earth and the stars at the same time. Responding to her mountain-like presence and steadiness, my autonomic nervous system "re-set" and my stress levels completely relaxed.

That experience of Anne as an immovable mountain – being so present and so balanced between heaven and earth – made a lasting impression on me. The feeling of her sitting beside me is still vivid in my memory. It lives on in my body and heart as a felt-sense memory of Anne's qualities of kindness, humility, total attentiveness, and groundedness: a state of being in which I could rest. I left with the hope that I also might be able to "set the stage" for my patients to have experiences like this. It was a great gift to me, and it is these qualities that I seek to bring to my practice more and more over time.

Connected to Earth

Caroline Tosh

Along with a few other osteopaths from the UK, I spent a wonderful day with Anne in her home. One of us had a bad cold and Anne took that opportunity to demonstrate her lymphatic drainage routine on him. In the process she really got that omentum wobbling!

Watching her give that treatment, I was struck by how grounded she was. When she sat down, you really got the sense of her being connected to the earth. It reminded me of what I had observed amongst those in the world who routinely squat in many of their daily actions – to me they seem to be more of the earth. There was this centeredness to all Anne's movements which came from this powerful, grounded, "seatedness." It was a striking experience – allowing me to really know just how grounded one could be.

My First Experiences

Caroline Tosh

My first exposure to Anne came at a basic course which was put on by the Sutherland Cranial Teaching Foundation in the UK in 1978. This was my first cranial course and a number of experiences with Anne really made a big impression on me. She was my table tutor on one of the days and I was struck by her presence. Her presence was warm; she was holding this open warmth which was not fussy at all. It made me think of a patient I had who was a nanny. When that nanny first came into my office, I had the feeling that it would be so nice to sit next to her. A feeling like you were at home. I felt it was the same with Anne.

During that day at the tables, when we were to do motion testing, I found that with her presence there was a spaciousness that made the perception much clearer. I remember sensing how the tide carried the tissues into the direction of ease, and how different that was to when you move to a barrier. I was able to discern the difference and to see that with the guidance of the tide I was not just moving tissue. It was my first instruction in letting the tissue show you what to do.

That same day, I observed Anne treating one of the students in our group who had been in an accident. As part of cutting down a tree, a chain was being winched, the chain snapped and ricocheted into her face – the force was tremendous. As I was watching Anne treat this young woman, I could see the shape of her face changing – like plastic being molded. You could see her complexion change from pasty gray back to normal; you could see her turning back into herself. It was quite amazing to me.

During that course, Anne also treated me for the effects of an injury. At the age of sixteen, in a swimming pool accident, I'd had a brain trauma and fracture of C1. It was this trauma that had led me to choose to go to osteopathic school. However, despite manipulative treatment from good and notable clinicians, I was still having a lot of neck trouble when Anne got hold of me. I remember she decompressed the cranial base and treated C1, and I felt pressure release and for the first time in seven years I could turn my neck without it getting stuck. The change was so dramatic that I was then inspired to learn all I could about cranial work and saw that it was what I really wanted to do thereafter. It was a pivotal experience.

Everybody's Here

Bonnie Gintis

There is something I heard Anne say at the start of some of the study group meetings that I appreciated. We would be sitting around, waiting for people to arrive, and she would take a look around the room and wait some more. Then a time would come when, even though several people were clearly missing, she would say "everybody's here" and start talking.

I felt like it was her way of acknowledging that whoever was there was *present* and she was going to begin with who was there. It wasn't about doing a head count, it seemed like her way of marking the moment in which it felt like the right time to start. It was a simple way of expressing the value of each person's attentiveness and presence and each person's place in a whole.

I Don't Know

Bonnie Gintis

I was always delighted with the many different ways in which Anne would say she did not know something. She might say she was "waiting for an answer" or "still exploring that." She seemed perfectly comfortable coming out and saying, "I don't know, but maybe someday I will." Or, she might say, "let's see if we can figure that out together." I always loved that aspect of studying with her; that honesty and joy in sharing what she did know and what she didn't know. I believe the biggest thing I got from Anne was seeing how she had taken the teaching she had received and integrated it into who she was. It supported my own desire to do the same for myself.

The Mechanism Reads Me

Andrew Goldman

For the developing osteopathic student, there is a natural tendency, as we learn to sense the involuntary mechanism in our patients, to search for it with our mind's eye. As I learned these osteopathic skills, I often found that table trainers would inform me that I was being too invasive. As I relinquished this intense, focused, *probing* method, I discovered that I would feel more and have a better sense of the patient's mechanism as it worked gracefully toward health. I became aware that I had been interfering with the mechanism's free motion, thereby inhibiting the full expression of corrective forces guided by the "Breath of Life."

This led to the idea that, although I could endeavor to search for the involuntary mechanism within the patient, it was much more fruitful to allow it to find me. This seemed to conflict with long-standing habits of diligent concentration that had always been rewarded with past success in a myriad of endeavors, academically and in other aspects of my life. As I tried to make sense of this conundrum, I had the good fortune to ask Anne Wales about it. I said, "It is my impression that the mechanism is reading *me* and assessing what I know, showing me what it needs *me* to do, how I would be most useful. It will even treat me during the process of treating the patient." I wanted to know if this was a reasonable thought or if, perhaps, I was misguided, even crazy. She answered simply, "I'm glad you know that that happens."

The Physical and the Spiritual

Maxwell Fraval

A colleague and I had the opportunity to spend a few
private hours with Anne Wales while attending a course
in New England in the 1990s. During that visit, she
spoke of some spiritual matters. She relayed a story from
another student of Sutherland's, Tom Schooley, in which
Dr. Schooley and an osteopathic colleague were at a lecture
given by the scientist-philosopher, Walter Russell. One of
them noted that he saw Russell as having a green light on
his forehead, which was interpreted by them as a sign of
spiritual development. Anne also told us of how she and
Dr. Sutherland had spoken about the experience of having
non-material guidance.

Hearing these stories from Anne and knowing that Walter
Russell and Dr. Sutherland had some connections – it
made me consider and deeply appreciate how Sutherland
was able to have deep knowledge of both the physical
and the spiritual. This was reassuring and re-enforcing for
me, as the potential for gaining both physical and inner
knowledge was an important motivation in my pursuit and
practice of osteopathy.

Present to the Natural World

Michael Burruano

My wife, Jeannene, and I picked Anne up at her home en route to the Sutherland Cranial Teaching Foundation Continuing Studies conference in Maine. The thing about that drive is that it goes through New Hampshire, which has state-owned liquor stores that do not charge a sales tax (which was 9% where we lived), and we had a coupon for an extra 10% discount. The annual trip to Maine was therefore enticing not only for the lessons to be learned at a great conference, but also to stock up on our wines and liquors for the year to come.

As we parked the car at the liquor store, I turned and asked Anne if she needed anything. Her reply? "A bottle of whiskey, please." I was not surprised by this; I loved the times I had shared with Anne over a glass of scotch or whiskey – times of great friendship and storytelling.

Anne waited in the car as Jeannene and I began our sojourn through the aisles of spirits and wines, and we quickly were lost in our task. When the task was completed, we were shocked to see it was forty-five minutes later. We returned to the car, ashamed to have left this 90-something-year-old beloved woman, friend, and teacher alone for so long in the back of our car.

We need not have worried. Upon our return we were greeted happily with this report: "From the position of the sun in the sky it is about 4:30 in the afternoon and from the contrails of the jets overhead I see that the winds are from the southwest and are fairly brisk..." and so it continued. It was a present-moment dissertation of the natural world and its workings. No moments wasted, no anticipation, simply recognition and being present to the constant background of the natural world: not just perception, but internalized cognition and knowing engagement, making the natural world her own – it a part of her and she a part of it.

An Infusion of Light

James Gaydos

In the early 2000s, a patient named "Janet" came to my office because she'd heard there was an osteopath in Montpelier, Vermont. She was in her mid-sixties and lived in a nearby city. Janet told me that her father was an osteopath who had lived in a rural town in Vermont from the 1930s to the 1950s. Her parents were hard-working folk from the Great Depression era who had found their way up to Vermont, from Rhode Island, looking for cheaper land and a better way of life. Her father worked long hours raising hay on a rented farm while working in town as an osteopath. I got the clear impression that these were not people accustomed to asking for help.

Janet grew up in that small town, married her high school sweetheart, then moved to find work and make a life together with her husband. When she came to me, some 40-plus years later, she was having a difficult time. Her husband had died suddenly and not long thereafter, her son and daughter-in-law had tragically died. Janet found herself increasingly isolated from her own feelings – full of pain from these losses and anxious about her future. Her daughter had invited her to move to Florida to be with family, but Janet felt immobilized. Her sadness was affecting her health and, not wishing to take the medication offered for her grief, she was delighted to see that there was an "old-fashioned osteopath" in Montpelier, and she was interested to see if this would help.

After she received the first of several treatments, Janet's curiosity was aroused, and she remarked that she "hadn't

been treated like that" since she was a girl. In reply to
her questions about how I was trained, I mentioned the
strong influence that an osteopath named Anne Wales had
made on my practice, as well as my life. I noted that the
room became silent...and that Janet had welled-up with
emotion. Something from long ago had stirred up a great
tide of memory within her, and she remained transfixed in
thought until, at last, she began to speak. Janet told me that
her parents had trouble conceiving and that she had been
adopted. It was a family secret that she'd long ago buried. Her
husband may have been the only other person, besides her
parents and their close friends, who knew this truth.

Then she told me the story of Anne's connection with her
family. Janet's father, "Doc," and Anne knew each other
through their osteopathic connections, and Anne would
come up to vacation with her family in Vermont to escape
the summer heat and crowded practice that she had in Rhode
Island. Anne had enjoyed these extended visits on the farm
where she could ride horses with Doc, discuss osteopathy, and
help out in the farm kitchen with Doc's wife. She was always
considered family.

It was during one of those visits that Anne heard of their
struggles to conceive. She then put out the word to her
colleagues letting them know of her Vermont "family's"
situation. News eventually returned of a child born in North
Carolina who was available for adoption. And so it was that

Anne and Janet's hopeful mother-to-be made the lengthy trip by train to meet and return home with Baby Janet.

Janet recalled receiving osteopathic treatments from Anne as a child and she too considered Anne as family. As time passed and she grew up and moved away, Janet grew more distant from her life in her hometown. Janet said she hadn't spoken to Anne in years and presumed that she was now deceased and was quite delighted to hear that Anne was alive and teaching. On a subsequent visit, she told me that she had called and spoken with Anne by telephone. It was a remarkable "reunion" that Janet and Anne shared, and that both delighted in recounting.

Ultimately, through the osteopathic care that she received, as well as a chance-of-a-lifetime reunion with Anne, Janet was restored in composure and health. She became confident in her decision to relocate to Florida to be with her daughter, and to start a new life as a grandmother.

Miracles in our lives occur when we least expect, brought to us by those whom we barely know, as well as by those whom we thought we knew. Anne was an infusion of light in my life and in the lives of so many others.

Step-by-Step

James Gaydos

I used to occasionally visit Anne in her trailer home in North Attleboro, seeking her perspective on osteopathy or for a treatment. On one occasion, it was to seek personal advice. Some events had occurred that left me frustrated, scared and angry. When I saw Anne, I didn't hold back. She listened intently for a while, before signaling me to get onto the treatment table.

During that treatment, her advice was sage: "Sometimes we find ourselves in a swamp, afraid to move, and with no known way out. It is then that we need to rely only on our sense that comes from each step; and then, step-by-step, we find our own way out of the mire."

Through the years, I have often thought of Dr. Wales' advice when meeting adverse conditions.

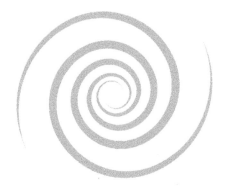

Don't Knead the Bread Too Much

Bonnie Gintis

My husband, Steve [Paulus], and I spent the first day of our honeymoon with Anne. She was especially delighted to welcome Steve and I that day as we were both about to turn 40 years old and Anne had married Chester Handy, DO around that same age, which was quite late in life for a woman in her time.

As part of the visit, we all treated each other. Steve had never met Anne before, so it was a particularly enlightening experience for him. As Steve and Anne had their hands on me, he was asking her about the many things he was feeling while the treatment happened. I can't remember exactly what Anne said, but the message we received was her telling us to beware that we don't think everything we feel is important and end up treating it all.

Anne explained that it is important to wait, because a lot of stuff will just come up, pass through, and ultimately not be important. She went on to say that if you start fiddling with everything that comes up it is like kneading the bread too much, the outcome is compromised. It also can obscure what is important. The big lesson for me that day was about just being patient during the treatment process. Anne was the embodiment of patience.

Waiting...

Caroline Tosh

In the 1980s, at what was probably my third Sutherland Cranial Teaching Foundation course in the UK, I had Anne as one of my table tutors. In a table session on directing the tide to the occipitomastoid suture, Anne showed us how to set up a diagonal oscillation and to sense the quality of the tide as it meets the restricted suture line. And then her instruction was just to wait until it becomes soft and still – for the oscillation to settle – before offering space to the suture. And then she instructed us to wait some more for the membranes to re-organize; and if you wait *well enough* (in distinction to long enough), you then have a change in the longitudinal fluctuation of the tide coming all the way up the patient that will move the suture. I don't think she used the term "well enough" but it is how I understood what she was saying and have always referred to it by that phrase.

In the decades since, I have often corrected students who think you can just send a bit of tide toward a suture and then spread it. It's actually a rather more exacting process as I learned it from Anne. Her demonstration taught me a lesson about patience. As I reflect back now on how Anne worked, my perception is that she really did work with the tissues synchronously with the fluid.

Reciprocal Tension

Richard Holding

In the early 1980s, after one of the cranial courses that Anne Wales taught in the UK, she stayed on with my wife and I for a few days. As part of that visit, we took a boat trip down the Thames River to Hampton Court and our major topic of conversation was reciprocal tension. She told a story of how one of Will's faculty was lecturing on the subject and described the ligaments as being stretched under reciprocal tension. Dr. Sutherland was in the classroom and turned to Anne and said, "ligaments don't get stretched, they change their shape."

As we continued down the Thames and came to the skyscrapers, we began an exercise in visualizing the shapes between the buildings, with Anne pointing out how, in the body, the reciprocal tension is actually in three dimensions. I remember her talking about a hanging mobile as a three-dimensional model for how there is a change in shape of the tissues when they lose connection to the master fulcrum. And so, as the body goes into disease, the shape changes.

We discussed the concept of all the organs and other tissues having an optimal shape to function normally. With treatment, allowing the area under our hands to find its Stillness and optimum shape within the reciprocal tension of the whole is our aim.

Snap to Attention

Rachel Brooks

Anne once came up to Boston to meet with a small group of us for a study session. I think it was in the late 1980s or early 90s. By that time, I had been treated by Anne many times over many years and was quite familiar with her hands and her approaches. But in that study session, I had a new experience.

Anne explained that she was going to demonstrate the procedure of testing for motion of the sphenobasilar synchondrosis. She asked for someone to lie down on the table, and I jumped at the chance to do so. Anne placed her hands on my vault with her usual firm and comfortable contact and spoke of what she observed. Then she said, "And now I am going to test for flexion;" and as she did, to my surprise, I clearly felt as if my tentorium cerebelli snapped downward into its full flexion position. Anne then observed my mechanism for a brief time as things returned to normal, and then she said: "And now I am going to test for extension." And, sure enough, I felt my tentorium make just as brisk a movement upward into its full extension position; it was like a soldier snapping to attention. Once again, she observed my mechanism settle back into its quiet rhythmic movement. Anne then declared that both of these tests showed normal, free movement and that was the end of that demonstration. I got off the table and felt perfectly fine – though still with a little wide-eyed surprise.

At that time, I already knew that it was very possible, and often quite helpful, to use active engagement and applied force when working with the mechanism, but I had never felt such a dramatic snap-to-attention type of input – in this case for diagnosis. That experience was a further reinforcement for me that we can actively engage with the mechanism without disturbing it if we are *working with* the mechanism and not just *doing things to* it. Anne and Rollin had both shown me that.

Rollin, even though he is most remembered for his attunement to Stillness and his fluid approach, almost always used some compressive forces in his treatments. The amount of compressive force was often mild, but it could be quite strong. His treatments had shown me that using active inputs did not require that he abandon either his awareness of Stillness or his use of fluids in order to "do things."

Anne used her hands in a firm way; they never felt too heavy, but they could be incredibly strong. During one treatment, I remember her decompressing my frontonasal suture and feeling her apply a good deal of force as she spread that compressed articulation. As always, she was very grounded and present while doing this. It certainly got my attention while she was exerting that force, though I felt no disturbance in my mechanism. After she was done, my face felt like it was two inches taller and that it had discovered a whole new open way of being. That got my attention too!

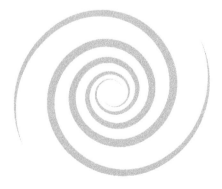

Anatomy Clear and Complete

Richard Holding

Dr. Wales really emphasized the necessity for accuracy in her anatomical view of what was happening beneath her hands. Once, when I was writing to get her opinion as to possible changes in the Sutherland Cranial Teaching Foundation courses being taught in the UK, she warned that whatever the expansion or addition of ideas there might be, it did not stop the need for the detailed study of the bones and sutures and their applied anatomy. She wrote back to me:

> Let me say that your problems with designing courses and conferences are the same as existed here all along. We do not have all the answers. By the time he [Will] had classes, he had organized his lectures to fit the profession at that time. Now that his teaching has been out in the world for so long, it may not be the best way to teach an Introductory Course. It is certainly not necessary. But somewhere along the way: *The anatomy must be clear and complete.* Otherwise, people will not know what they are doing in diagnosis and treatment.

I have taken this message very much to heart in my own teaching over the years.

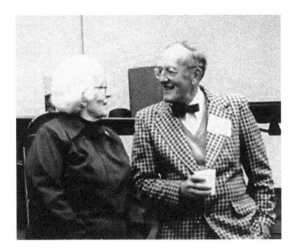
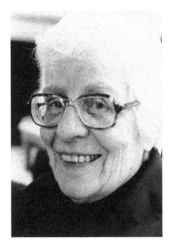

Dr. Wales and Dr. Becker during the 1980 SCTF course at the West Virginia College of Osteopathic Medicine. Photos by Mark Rosen, DO.

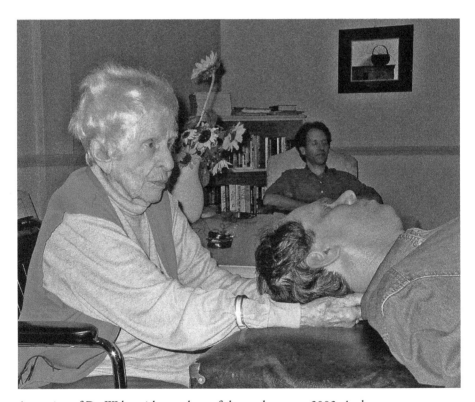

A meeting of Dr. Wales with members of the study group, 2003. Andrew Goldman is being treated. In the background is Donald Hankinson who remarked, "I am in a state of blissful repose, having just been treated by Anne."

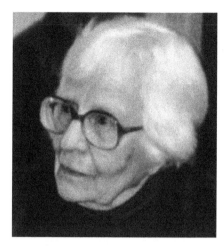

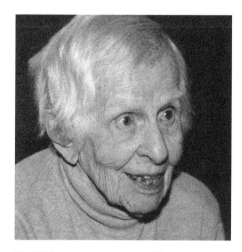

Dr. Wales listening to a discussion in the anatomy lab at the University of New England College of Osteopathic Medicine. Cropped image of a photo by Andrew Haltof, DO.

Dr. Wales at 100 years old. Photo by Henry Nield/Sue Turner, DO.

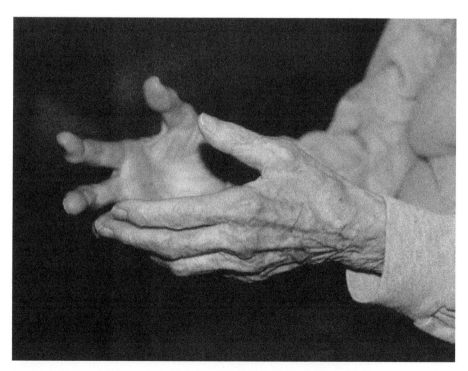

The hands of Dr. Wales at 100. Photo by Henry Nield/Sue Turner, DO.

On This Frontier

Michael Burruano

In 1996, members of the "A Still-Sutherland Study Group," that had been meeting with Anne for some years, were about to start a teaching program. My memory is that she had told us it was time to get on with it and teach what she was teaching us, and so we did. It was a wonderful time – we were exploding with enthusiasm and growth. Anne was using Will's words with us, but unlike many others, she used them as a means of studying and exploring past a preconceived endpoint.

On the eve of that ASSSG course, Anne sent me a letter that included this passage:

> The point that appears every now and then is that even the Osteopathic Profession does not see the magnitude of the Science of Osteopathy. That is, we really are on a frontier. If anyone thinks that this subject is all wrapped up and ready to teach, they are not "in the know." This is one fact that makes life on this frontier so exciting: There is always something to be learned.

Over the years, when teaching the study group, Anne patiently repeated what Dr. Sutherland had taught her and what she had learned. Those in any generation who thought they had it "all wrapped up" were not new to her, and her response to them was always the same. She would say, "All you can do is put the truth out there, but you can't do anything about what people do with it." Having received the gift of these teachings from her, I know for a fact that there is always something to be learned.

Passing on Sutherland's Teaching

Michael Burruano

One of Anne's great gifts to us was the dedication she had to passing on with care and dutiful accuracy what she had been given by Dr. Sutherland. While he was alive, Dr. Sutherland was determined to make sure that the cranial concept he had developed was taught properly. It was the result of fifty years of work and he knew it was probable that he would die before saying all he had to say. So, he needed there to be clear teaching of *his* concept. Therefore, according to Anne, when a lecturer veered from the point in a basic course, his exclamation of, "That is not what I am trying to say," was not so much an admonishment, but a clarification.

When students of Sutherland approached him for confirmation of their understanding of a part of the concept, he would often reply, "keep digging." Apparently, some took this in a negative context, but Anne saw this reply as one of support and encouragement. In the same way, when students and colleagues would offer thoughts and explorations for discussion with Anne, her frequent response was: "That is not what Dr. Sutherland was trying to say." To me, this was not meant to be demeaning or dismissive of their idea, but only a reminder of her mission to give her students sight of what Dr. Sutherland was teaching. I took from this the notion that it is good to keep digging and learning, but it is also important to keep clear what Sutherland was teaching and pointing to.

Harry…an Anne Tale

Michael Burruano

While sitting in the living room of her home, Anne related the story of how her husband, Chester, had once cared for cloistered nuns whose monastery was nearby. He would travel there and have a room to work in to treat the sisters. She told us how, after Vatican II, some breath was given for the sisters to travel and with the passing of Chester, Anne had taken over the duty and they would come to see her. One day she received a frantic call telling her that Harry was unable to move his legs, was in great distress and could they bring him right over. Anne said, "Yes." Much to Anne's surprise, three nuns showed up with Harry – their pet rabbit – who seemed in a bad way with an injured back. In true Anne style, she relayed how she studied the situation and decided that she did, indeed, know something about the spine of vertebrates, and so she sat on the couch with Harry in her lap and began to palpate and examine the situation.

Meanwhile, it should be understood that Harry was dear to these nuns and their anxiety was at a peak. Anne painted a picture of her on the couch with the sisters pacing quickly, frantically, without purpose, back and forth behind the couch and around the room while she sat quietly focused on Harry. She found a point of balanced tension in the involved area and therapeutics got to work. Anne looked up in telling the story and said, "Did you ever notice how sometimes during a treatment the whole room goes still?"

I love the mental picture of the frantically pacing nuns and Anne, with Harry, in the center of the couch with stillness pervading the room. After a time, Harry got up and began to hop about, and I have carried the image of the Still in the midst of the Frantic/the Motion as a lesson and an analogy for many years both personally and professionally.

Not Beholden to the Clock

Mary Bayno

I started dancing at the age of five. I danced ballet, jazz, and modern styles semi-professionally for 25 years by the time my very wide feet and I met Anne. By then I had chronic pain in my right foot and had to be careful about which shoes I wore. My podiatric exam and x-rays were normal (although one podiatrist told me that my EE wide feet had enough room between the first and second toes to fit in another toe). Lucky for me, in the year I met Anne she was teaching the study group her balanced ligamentous approach to treating the feet. I was intrigued. At school I remembered only being taught one single high velocity technique for the foot.

During a subsequent visit with Anne, I asked her to take a look at my right foot. She started by addressing my pelvis using the "differential technique," which is what she always did with me. Then, having sorted my pelvis and ribs out, she moved down to my tibiofibular interosseous membrane. Finally, after examining my right foot, Anne said, "Well, I know what the problem is. Your right cuboid has dropped."

To treat this, she shifted my leg so that my foot was off the table, took hold of my fourth and fifth metatarsals and let the foot dangle. She said that gravity would carry the calcaneus away from the cuboid and the cuboid away from the fourth and fifth metatarsals, and this would create the space necessary for the cuboid to resume its normal position in the lateral longitudinal arch. And then she held the foot that way for 45 minutes!

The reason I know it was 45 minutes is this: Typically, during a treatment, Anne chatted. She would chat about her life, Dr. Still or Dr. Sutherland, her patients, or anything else that came to mind. One of her favorite topics with me was to describe the train routes she took from Tiverton, Rhode Island to Kirksville, Missouri in her journey to osteopathic school as a very young adult. I often found myself falling asleep as she talked and treated – and that day I had quickly slipped into that trance-like state. Then, as Anne began examining the foot the big clock she had chimed; the chime woke me and I heard her make her diagnosis. I was awake as she began to dangle my foot, but then she resumed her talk of trains and I promptly fell asleep again.

The next thing I knew, I was startled awake by Anne saying, "Well, now your cuboid has repositioned itself into its proper place." I looked at the clock – 45 minutes had passed. She had patiently dangled my foot for 45 minutes. Anne used to say that the good thing about retirement was that she was no longer beholden to the clock.

My right foot has been pain-free ever since, and for 30 years I have tried to provide the same relief to my patients whether they danced or not.

A Perfect Bite

James Gaydos

I had a practice in Lee County, Florida, from 1994 to 1999, and my first office was located not far from the vantage point where Sutherland observed the effect of the tide upon the Caloosahatchee River[1]. My second office was on Sanibel Island, an area possibly known to Dr. Sutherland for his observations of shell-pickers[2]. As many New Englanders vacationed and retired along the gulf coast, there were patients of Dr. Wales who sought me out in their search for osteopathic care. These patients' stories provided the subject matter for the many phone conversations that I shared with Dr. Wales through those years.

One patient was a 15-year-old girl, brought in by her parents with an earache. The father said that they had been seen by an osteopath in New England, where they had moved from several years before, and wanted her to be treated in order to avoid the use of antibiotics. During the examination and treatment, I remarked that their daughter had the most remarkably perfect bite, and that I was surprised that I could sense no strain within her as a result the orthodontic work I presumed she must have had. An exchange with her father followed:

Dad: "That's because she never had braces – she was treated by an osteopath."
Me: "Really? That's remarkable. Who did she treat with?"
Dad: "You wouldn't know her. She's dead."
Me: "Hmm...but what was her name?"
Dad: "Her name was Anne Wales."
Me: "Oh, I know Anne. She's not dead; she just wrote a book!"[3]

[1] *Teachings in the Science of Osteopathy,* p. 15.
[2] *Contributions of Thought,* Fascial Drag and the Fulcrum; 1st ed. p. 197, 2nd ed. p. 283.
[3] Anne Wales was the editor of *Teachings in the Science of Osteopathy.*

A Reminder to Think Osteopathy

James Gaydos

The father of one of my patients, who was a karate enthusiast, came into my office on occasion. One time he mentioned Dr. Wales and told me of the history of the care he had received from her. The man had been involved in an accident where he rolled his truck. Luckily, he had escaped largely unharmed, except that his hand had gone through the windshield with resulting fractures, edema, and ecchymosis.

He was seen at the local emergency room where the attending orthopedist sent him home simply with instructions to ice his hand. The doctor told him there was too much swelling to cast or even splint the hand, and they couldn't discuss surgery until the massive edema had cleared. Hearing this, the gentleman immediately called Anne, who told him to come over.

I later spoke to Dr. Wales about the remarkable response he had under her care. As Anne recalled, "there wasn't much that I could do for him, except open the lymphatic channels in the neck, thoracic inlet and affected forearm." But then, sitting quietly and holding his hand she had an idea. She proceeded to slowly introduce the back of her own hand into the palm of the man's very swollen hand; and then she used the natural curvature of her hand to support his hand and apply individual traction to each metacarpal and digit, thereby treating each fractured structure. Dr. Wales did this on a regular basis, eventually substituting the placement of a tennis ball into the man's hand so that she could use both hands in her work.

The end result was "very satisfying" according to Dr. Wales. The man told me he never had to have surgery and had remained free from pain to the point where he was free to use his hand in all his usual activities, including being able to make a full fist and pursue his studies in karate. I kept a tennis ball on my office desk for many years in memory of Anne's words, and for the reminder to "Think Osteopathy" – a phrase Dr. Sutherland used in instruction to his students.

Can Treat Anything

Anthony Norrie

Once, when I was visiting in New England at a Sutherland Cranial Teaching Foundation conference, I had a chance to spend some time with Anne. During that visit she told a story of how she had a man come to her for treatment of his hand that had multiple fractures. He had been involved in some trauma, was a martial artist, and did not want to go down the surgical treatment route proposed at the emergency room. Anne recounted how she thought for a time about how she could possibly treat this severely swollen hand and how to do it without causing more pain for the man or more trauma to the tissues.

She explained she did this by letting the man rest his curled hand on top of her relaxed fist, allowing her to gently contact the PRM. She described how she just sat and waited until she felt the expression of the PRM move into the hand, at which point she removed hers, replaced it with a tennis ball and bandaged the hand around it. Anne then related how the man had returned for more treatment and after some time all his fractures completely resolved with no deformity or other sequelae.

At that time this story was a big encouragement to me in my practice skills, and I have used this notion many times in practice. I have seen fractures successfully reduced doing nothing else. More importantly, I also came away with the understanding that I could try to treat anything that might present itself, even if I was uncertain of the outcome. Using Anne's lesson, I saw that by simply getting the mechanism going, really positive results could unfold.

I Can't Help You

Rachel Brooks

One day, early in my practice life in the mid-1980's, during one of my regular visits with Anne, she was telling me of a patient she had seen. I don't remember many of the details, but what I do remember was her conclusion that she had decided she could not help this person. As I recall, part of the reason was that her osteopathic treatments were not having an appreciable effect, and part of it had to do with some obstacle she felt in the patient or maybe in her relationship with them. I clearly remember her saying that it was OK to tell a patient you cannot help them; though she made it clear to me that she would never say "Osteopathy can't help you." Instead, she would say, "*I* can't help you."

One of the meanings this had for me at the time was to understand that there could be many reasons why you might choose not to engage with or continue with a patient. However, the really big lesson for me was the insight that choosing not to help someone was not synonymous with being uncaring or a failure. It helped me to understand the multi-layered reality of our relationships with patients and that even if they wanted to stay on, it was OK for me to say, "no." Even though I learned this lesson from Anne early in my career, for me it was a long-term work-in-progress to rest comfortably with this idea and be able to speak these often-difficult truths to patients. It took me 30-plus years to be able to do this with the true level of assurance and clarity that Anne had demonstrated that day.

Figure It Out For Yourself

Rachel Brooks

Over a span of seven years in the 1980s, Anne and I worked together to produce the book of Dr. Sutherland's teachings, *Teachings in the Science of Osteopathy*. Amongst the many challenges in the project was the necessity of editing Sutherland's spoken words into written words, in a clear way that strictly maintained his meaning. One of the tasks given to me was to read through Anne's initial manuscript and point to those places where we might consider making changes; to point out passages that read roughly or where the meaning was muddied by grammar and wording issues.

There were a number of places in which Anne accepted, sometimes with modification, my suggested changes in wording or phrasing. There were also a few places where she wanted the text to remain unchanged, and one of those places Anne wanted to leave unchanged really bothered me. I brought that passage to Anne's attention more than once – pointing out the lack of clarity. Finally, I said something like, "Anne, people are not going to understand what Sutherland meant; there will be confusion." To which she replied emphatically, "Well, *I* do not know what he meant, and each person is going to have to figure it out for themselves; each person will need to make of it what they will."

For me, this was a strong lesson in the power of personal honesty; it said so much about Anne's integrity as a purveyor of Will's teachings. Anne often said that she was not concerned about what people made of Dr. Sutherland's work. But what she did mind and could not abide was when people said, "This is what Will said" or "This is what Will meant," when she knew he neither said nor meant that. In this situation of the text in the book that I was asking her to change, she knew what Will had said but she did not know what he meant, and so she left the text as it was.

This exchange was hugely important to me, particularly as I was in my early days of teaching with the Sutherland Cranial Teaching Foundation in that same time period. As a result, from the very start of my teaching endeavors, I have believed it to be a matter of principle and care for me to be really clear about representing what my teachers had taught me. To clearly distinguish between: what my teachers had literally said; what *their* interpretation of it was if they had shared it with me; and what *my* interpretation was, then or now, of what they had said.

Anne's statement also helped me by letting me know it was OK not to understand it all and it was OK to come to my own conclusions. She also gave me the picture that we are all on an osteopathic path and we all are called upon to "dig on." And, where each of us goes with our digging will not, and probably can not or should not, be the same.

Students Forever

Zina Pelkey

As a student, I was privileged to attend a birthday party for Anne when she was in her late 80's. After the lobsters and birthday cake, Andy Haltof projected some slides on a huge screen for Anne's next presentation. One of the pictures was of the articulation of the frontal bone with the maxilla (Anne would say: It hangs like a tea ball from the frontal). In this slide the area was greatly enlarged so we could see the interdigitations in excellent detail. Anne jumped out of her chair and started bouncing up and down on her feet like a child at Christmas saying, "Oh! Oh! Now I will be able to treat that!"

My take-home message from her response was that we are all students forever – and I saw how satisfying and fun that could be.

A Developing Embryo

Donald Hankinson

In 1995, I was discussing with Dr. Wales
my plan to begin my upcoming lecture
on the face at the Sutherland Cranial
Teaching Foundation Basic Course, with its
embryologic development. I asked her if she
felt that would be appropriate. "Well," she
said, "When does that process that starts at
conception stop? Does the adult form finish
the process? I am 91 years old and I'm still
a developing embryo. I think that's kind of
a good picture. It's breathtaking!" Anne was
ever the developing embryo, embracing life
open-heartedly, respecting and cherishing all
within it. She modelled that it was possible
for all of us to do so with passion, humility,
and a sense of humor.

This was not just a poetic thought for Dr.
Wales, she lived it. In 2001, when Anne
turned 97 years old, the study group asked her
what she would like for a present. And, true
to form, Anne said that she would like a new
physiology text. A few weeks later, Andrew
Haltof stopped by her house for a visit and
found Anne sitting on her porch reading
the new textbook. Later, as she was treating
him, she reviewed what she had learned

reading about the negative pressures in the interstitium and the changes in that pressure as the lymphatic fluid moved through the lymphatic system. Then she paused, and said "Gee, if I'd only known that 50 years ago!"

Later that month, Dr. Wales came to our next study group meeting with a page of notes on what she had learned about the lymphatic system, complete with a page of diagrams illustrating the anatomy and physiology of the interface between the capillaries and the terminal lymphatics. Anne told us, "I learned something about the lymphatics after reading my new physiology text and my treatments have been so much better!" And, as she said this, I could feel the whole group let out a huge sigh of relief: if Anne was still learning at 97 years old, there was the opportunity for all of us to do the same. If we could keep our minds and hearts as open as Dr. Wales had done, like her, each of us could also realize our birthright as a developing embryo.

Outlive Them

Caroline Tosh

I spent a day with Anne in her home in 1990, and during that visit
I mentioned to her my experience of how the osteopathic profession
in the UK were regarding cranial work – how this work is not always
popular and there are people who don't agree with it and say we should
not do it. I knew that in her time there was also a fair amount of
criticism from the profession in the US and I wondered how she had
managed that. In response, Anne straightened herself up and said,
"There are those people who have not always agreed with my point of
view; many of them are no longer here." The message I took away from
this is that we just need to persevere – to keep doing what we believe
in and what we see work so well. And, if we can, live long enough to
outlast the critics just as Anne did.

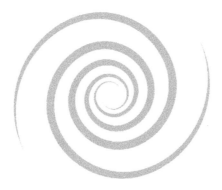

Anne Waking Up

Michael Burruano

One day in November 2002, Andrew Haltof, Tim Kingsbury, and I went to visit Anne Wales at the nursing home. She was asleep when we arrived. She slowly opened her eyes, looked up and said, "Oh, there's something I want to tell you…." She then began: "The jugular vein passes through the jugular fossa and drains from the sigmoid sinus which become the transverse sinus at the articulation of the inferior posterior angle of the parietal bone on the mastoid portion of the temporal…." She continued this tour of the venous drainage of the brain and fluid fluctuation in the cranium for what seemed like 20 to 40 minutes while we quietly listened.

We watched, and her appearance changed, waking up a bit at a time, as she seemed to be flicking on switches in her brain as she moved from brainstem to cortex through the living anatomy. At the end, now "fully awake," she looked up and spoke in her familiar sparkling voice that reflected her sincere joy in friendship and hospitality, "Oh, Andrew, Tim, Michael, it is so good to see you!"

Anne was amazing. How did she do that?! The words she recited came from the carefully recorded notes of Rebecca Lippincott, but the lesson came from the *soul and being* of Anne Wales – from a place that was present before she was. That presence manifests the heart and wise countenance in the face of Will Sutherland – a teaching directed from Still and received by Will's faculty. I have felt grateful and humbled to be a part of that lineage.

Anne Departing

Mary Bayno

I want to share my story of Anne's death. She was such an important person in my life. I first connected with Anne as a new physician in 1990 and maintained a treasured relationship until her death 15 years later. For me, as for many others, Anne was teacher – colleague – friend – mother/grandmother.

In the last few years of her life, Anne resided in a nursing facility as her physical capacities were gradually failing. Many of us who were closely connected to Anne, continued to keep an eye on her, and in the months before her death she was clearly going down. Despite her decline, she was still enthusiastic and happy to see all who came to visit.

Then, one day I received a call from someone who had recently seen her saying that Anne's legs were not working. It wasn't apparent to this person that she had suffered a stroke, but something was going on. When I heard this, I felt pretty certain that Anne was dying and thought somebody should be there. So, I got on the ferry near my home on Long Island and went to her bedside. There, I found Anne with the labored breathing of someone in the early stages of dying. Her eyes were closed, and I saw that her lips and tongue were very dry.

I spoke to Anne, telling her who I was and asked if I could give her a bit of thickened water. She did not speak but opened her eyes and looked clearly into my eyes and blinked. And so, I gave her bits of water over the next four hours.

Sitting there, the room was filled with a sacred stillness as she continued her slow labored breathing, which was rhythmic and peaceful. Anne's breathing seemed much more deliberate than the breathing of the other dying patients I had been with. It struck me that what I was seeing was her actively doing the work of dying, giving birth to herself in reverse. She was laboring, with determination and without fear, in what seemed to be a birthing process, transforming herself from this life into what came next. I knew, from long conversations with Anne, that she was certain death was not the end of existence.

In those hours at her bedside, I sat in a privileged silence while stroking her limp hand – memorizing its veins, contours, and Heberden's nodes. Those amazing hands! I told her how much I loved her and would miss her. Unexpectedly her hand gave mine a squeeze. She had heard me.

Eventually, I saw it was time for me to leave to catch the last ferry home. Overcome with emotion at saying my final goodbye, I began to sob – loud, messy sobs. Suddenly Anne opened her eyes, stared at me hard, concerned. I reassured her that I was fine; just so sad that I would not see her again. She closed her eyes and returned to her work. I marveled that Anne had any control in this death process, exiting briefly a second time in order to be of service to me. I felt remorse that I had interrupted her but awed by the gift of seeing it done.

In the few days that followed, others deeply connected with her stayed by her bedside until she departed, at the age of 101½.

I think people should know that Anne died the way she lived: fully present, focused, patient, and generous.

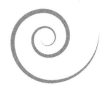

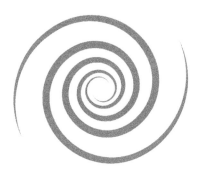

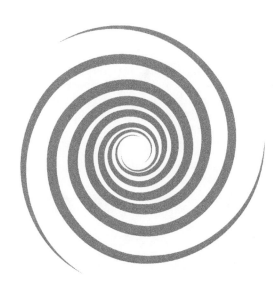

List of Contributors

Mark Baker, DO graduated from the European School of Osteopathy, United Kingdom, in 1992. He practices in France.

Mary S. Bayno, DO, C-SPOMM graduated from the University of New England College of Osteopathic Medicine in 1987.

Rachel E. Brooks, MD, FCA graduated from the University of Michigan Medical School in 1979.

Michael P. Burruano, DO, FCA graduated from the Philadelphia College of Osteopathic Medicine in 1982.

David J. Douglas-Mort, DO, BA, PG.Dip.CrO graduated from the British School of Osteopathy in 1976.

Jacques A. Duval, DO graduated from the British School of Osteopathy in 1963. He practiced in France.

Paula L. Eschtruth, DO, FCA graduated from the Chicago College of Osteopathic Medicine in 1964.

Maxwell Fraval, DO, M.Osteo.Sc (Paediatrics) graduated from the British School of Osteopathy in 1978 with further training in Australia. He practices in Australia.

James E. Gaydos, DO graduated from the University of New England College of Osteopathic Medicine in 1985.

Bonnie Gintis, DO graduated from the New York College of Osteopathic Medicine in 1986.

Andrew Goldman, DO, FCA graduated from the University of New England College of Osteopathic Medicine in 1989.

Nicholas Handoll, DO graduated from the British School of Osteopathy in 1971.

Donald Hankinson, DO graduated from the New York College of Osteopathic Medicine in 1985.

Richard Holding, DO graduated from the British School of Osteopathy in 1969.

Richard W. Koss, DO graduated from the Kirksville College of Osteopathic Medicine in 1982.

Christopher Laseter, DO, AOBNMM graduated from the Kirksville College of Osteopathic Medicine in 1990.

R. Paul Lee, DO, FAAO, FCA graduated from the University of Health Sciences, College of Osteopathic Medicine in Kansas City in 1976.

Thomas M. McCombs, DO, C-FP, C-NMMOMM graduated from the Oklahoma State University College of Osteopathic Medicine in 1987.

Anthony Norrie, DO graduated from the European School of Osteopathy, United Kingdom, in 1986. He practices in New Zealand.

Zinaida Pelkey, DO, FCA graduated from the New York College of Osteopathic Medicine in 1992.

Caroline Penn, DO, MSc(Ost), FSCCO, PHI (Handle Inst) graduated from the British School of Osteopathy in 1979.

Thomas Thrall, MD graduated from the Indiana University School of Medicine in 1979.

Caroline A. Tosh, DO, MSc, FSCCO graduated from the British School of Osteopathy in 1978.

Susan Turner, DO graduated from the European School of Osteopathy, United Kingdom, in 1979.

Patrick Wedlake, DO graduated from the University of North Texas Health Science Center (Texas College of Osteopathic Medicine) in 1987. He practices in the USA and Chile.

FCA: Fellow of the Cranial Academy
FSCCO: Fellow of the Sutherland Cranial College of Osteopathy

Books Cited

Becker, Rollin E. *Life in Motion: The Osteopathic Vision of Rollin E. Becker, DO.* Edited by Rachel E. Brooks, Stillness Press, 1997.

Becker, Rollin E. *The Stillness of Life: The Osteopathic Philosophy of Rollin E. Becker, DO.* Edited by Rachel E. Brooks, Stillness Press, 2000.

Eiseley, Loren. *The Immense Journey.* Originally published 1957.

Fulford, Robert C. *Are We on the Path? The Collected Works of Robert C. Fulford, DO, FCA.* Edited by Theresa A. Cisler, The Cranial Academy, 2003.

Fulford, Robert C. *Dr. Fulford's Touch of Life.* Written with Gene Stone, Pocket Books, 1996.

Handoll, Nicholas. *The Anatomy of Potency: Energy Osteopathy and Quantum Physics,* 2nd ed., Osteopathic Supplies, 2016.

Lee, R. Paul. "Palpation: Electric or Magnetic." *The Cranial Letter,* 2017, Osteopathic Cranial Academy. Available on Dr. Lee's website: cranialosteopathy.com.

Russell, Walter. *The Divine Iliad, 2 Volumes.* Originally published 1949.

Still, Andrew T. *Philosophy of Osteopathy.* American Academy of Osteopathy. Originally published 1899.

Still, Andrew T. *Osteopathy Research and Practice.* American Academy of Osteopathy. Originally published 1910.

Sutherland, William G. *Contributions of Thought: The Collected Writings of William Garner Sutherland, DO.* Edited by Adah Strand Sutherland and Anne L. Wales, 2nd ed., Sutherland Cranial Teaching Foundation, 1998.

Sutherland, William G. *Teachings in the Science of Osteopathy.* Edited by Anne L. Wales, Sutherland Cranial Teaching Foundation, 1990.

About the Editor

Rachel E. Brooks, MD

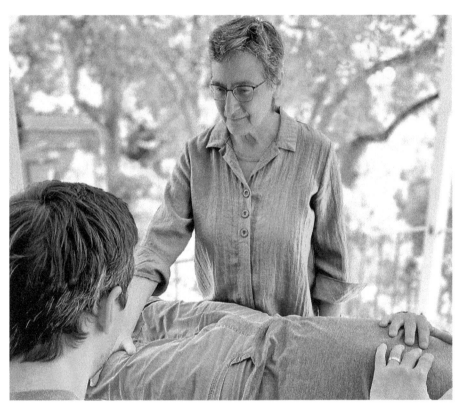

Dr. Rachel Brooks teaching her Power of Presence course in Portland, Oregon, 2022.

Dr. Brooks' lifelong dedication to osteopathy began when she met Rollin E. Becker, DO in 1975, just as she was entering the University of Michigan Medical School. Dr. Becker, a great practitioner and teacher of "cranial osteopathy," had been a close student of Dr. WG Sutherland, the founder of that osteopathic approach. After graduating from medical school and completing a residency in physical medicine and rehabilitation, Dr. Brooks moved to Boston and there she began her private practice in osteopathy in 1983. Living in New England

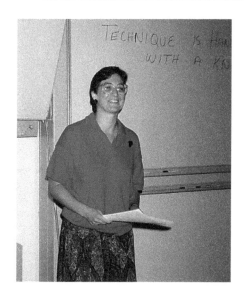

Dr. Rachel Brooks teaching at an SCTF course in the 1990s. On the board, partially seen, she has written a quote from Dr. Edna Lay: "Technique is hand placement together with a thorough knowledge of the mechanism."

for 11 years, she also had the opportunity to study closely with Anne L. Wales, DO, another dedicated student of Dr. Sutherland's.

Dr. Brooks has been teaching cranial osteopathy since 1986 and served as a member of the board of trustees of the Sutherland Cranial Teaching Foundation for sixteen years, from 1988–2004. Over the years, she has taught post-graduate courses across the US and internationally; and Dr. Brooks continues to be sought worldwide for her personal and historical insights regarding the practice and foundations of osteopathic practice. She currently teaches a series of courses titled, "The Power of Presence."

In addition to her teaching, Dr. Brooks has undertaken a number of publication projects. Her initial editorial effort, in the 1980s, was to assist Anne Wales, DO in the editing of *Teachings in the Science of Osteopathy* by William G. Sutherland, DO, and she helped edit the second edition of Sutherland's *Contributions of Thought*. In 1997, she founded Stillness Press.

Rachel E. Brooks, MD is the editor of these Stillness Press books:

- *Life in Motion: The Osteopathic Vision of Rollin E. Becker, DO*
- *The Stillness of Life: The Osteopathic Philosophy of Rollin E. Becker, DO*
- *Three Great Teachers of Osteopathy: Lessons We Learned from Drs. Becker, Fulford, and Wales.*

Information about Stillness Press books is available at: **stillnesspress.com**

Printed in the USA
CPSIA information can be obtained
at www.ICGtesting.com
LVHW061758030124
768084LV00058B/1238